THE

EASY FITNESS WORKBOOK

THE

EASY FITNESS WORKBOOK

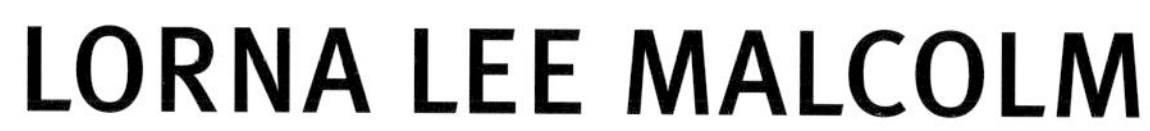

LORNA LEE MALCOLM

DUNCAN BAIRD PUBLISHERS
LONDON

The Easy Fitness Workbook
Lorna Lee Malcolm

First published in the United Kingdom
and Ireland in 2005 by
Duncan Baird Publishers Ltd
Sixth Floor
Castle House
75–76 Wells Street
London W1T 3QH

Conceived, created and designed by
Duncan Baird Publishers

Managing Editor: Julia Charles
Editor: Zoë Stone
Managing Designer: Manisha Patel
Designer: Justin Ford

British Library Cataloguing-in-Publication Data:
A CIP record for this book is available from the British Library

ISBN-10: 1-84483-080-2
ISBN-13: 9-781844-83080-0

10 9 8 7 6 5 4 3 2 1

Typeset in TradeGothic
Colour reproduction by Colourscan, Singapore
Printed in China by Imago

NOTES
Before following any advice or practice suggested in this book, it is recommended that you consult your doctor as to its suitability, especially if you suffer from any health problems or special conditions. The publisher, the author and the photographer cannot accept any responsibility for any injuries or damage incurred as a result of following the exercises in this book, or of using any of the therapeutic techniques described or mentioned here.

To Granny and Grandad Nichols.
We miss you Grandad, but know you are watching over us.

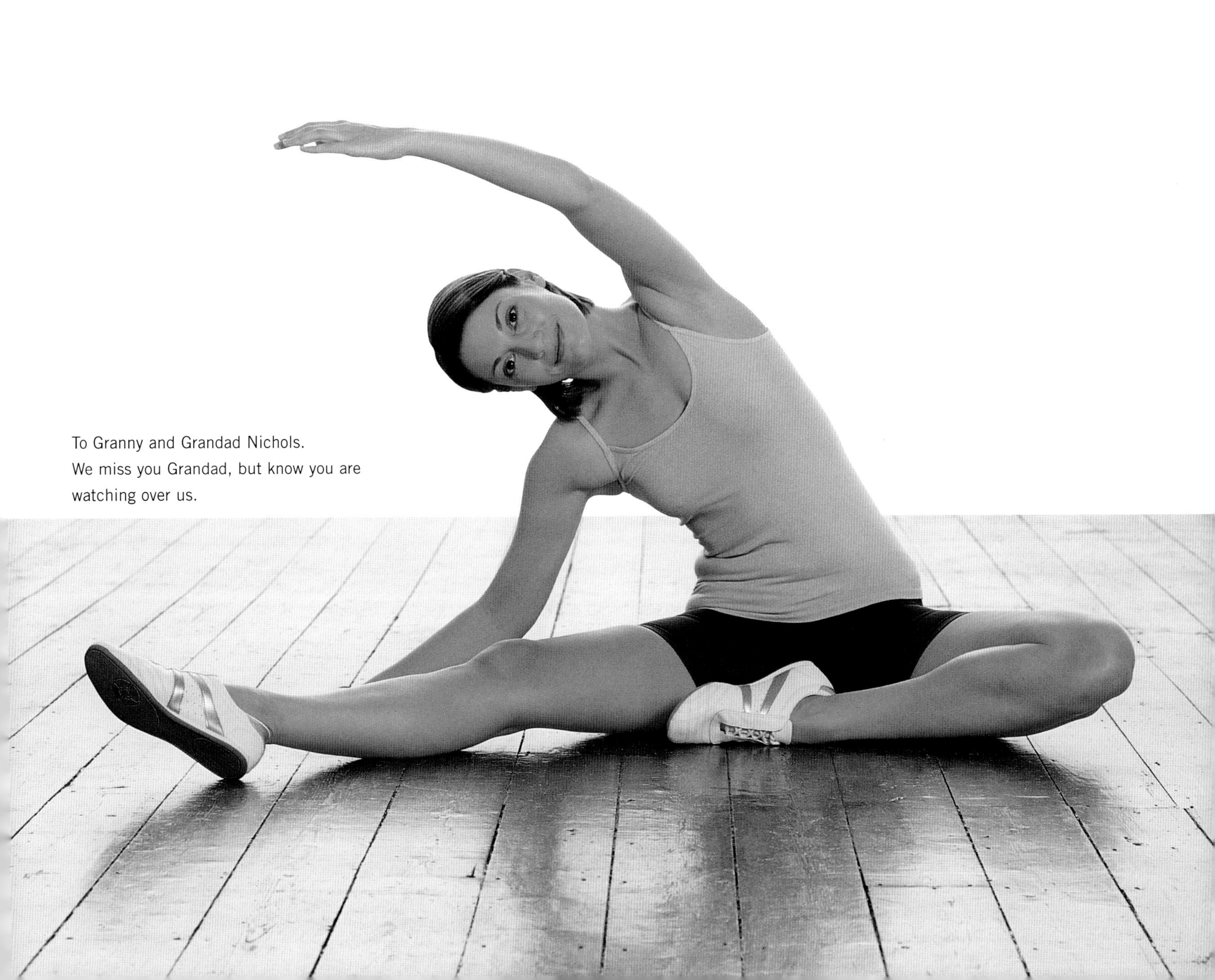

Contents

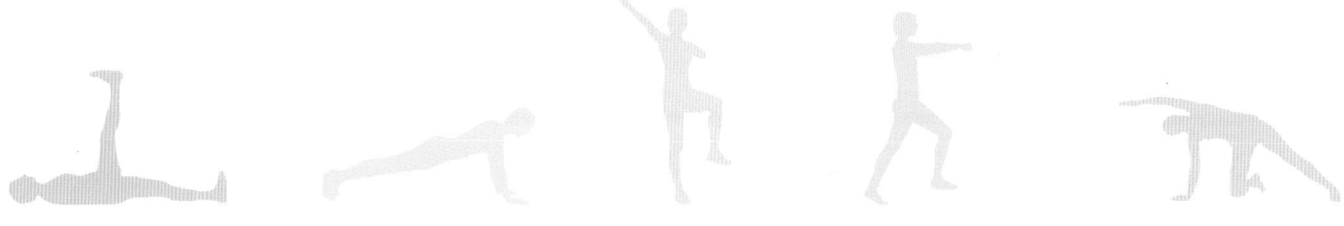

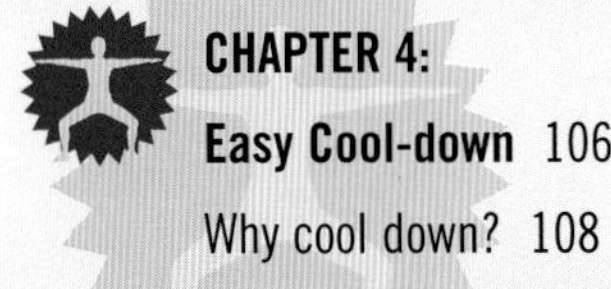

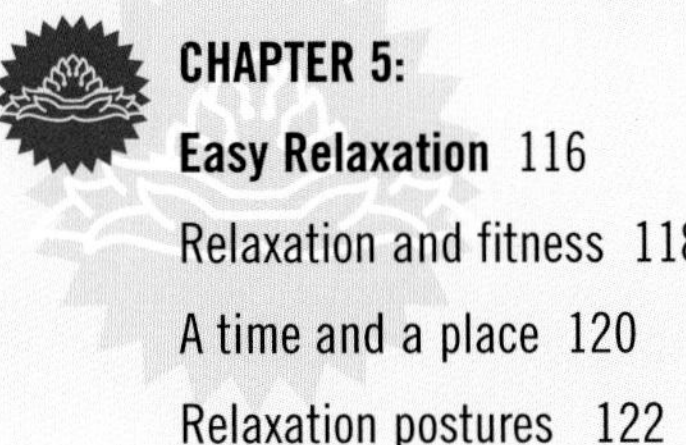

SYMBOLS USED IN THIS BOOK

- **3** — **CD track number**
- ✓ — **Exercise is good for ... / Solution to problem**
- ✗ — **Avoid if ... / Problem with exercise**
- ! — **Take care if you suffer from ...**
- ◎ — **See Chapter 3 for troubleshooting tips**

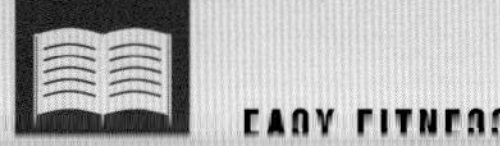

Author's introduction

This is my fourth book in eight years. In that time there has been only a small increase in the number of people who are health club members, despite all the media and promotional information that is constantly generated about the benefits of being more physically active.

The health club figures do not take account of the number of people who, for whatever reason, cannot or do not wish to join a health club, but do regularly exercise and have increased their levels of daily physical activity over the years. If you are already physically active or thinking about becoming so, and wish to work out at home rather than in a club or centre, this book is for you.

I passionately feel that healthy levels of physical activity should be an integral part of every person's life in the same way that eating, drinking and sleeping is essential to life. As I get older (46 next birthday!) I appreciate the benefits that fitness gives me more and more every day. I approach working out with a joyous mental attitude because it helps me to be positive, enjoy what I do and reap mental as well as physical benefits. Of course there are times when doing the exercises is tough, time is against me or I temporarily lack the necessary energy or motivation, but I know that once I start exercising the endorphins will start flowing and my energy levels will rise. At the end of the workout I will feel a sense of achievement and well-being and I can give myself a pat on the back for completing as much as I can do on any particular day and investing in my future quality of life.

I wish everyone the gift of life-long mobility and hope that using my book will contribute to this.

How to use this book

This book is a class within a book and contains all you will need for a total body workout, which includes exercises that target and improve elements of your cardiovascular, muscular, nervous and skeletal systems.

• Chapter 1 introduces you to the benefits of physical fitness activity. It tells you what "fitness" actually is and gives you some useful information that will help clarify why you are doing the exercises included. This chapter also comprises the warm-up.

• Chapter 2 contains the workout format that is the same as any workout you would do in a leisure centre or health club save that you can do it in the privacy and comfort of your own home. There are cardiovascular exercises, followed by a strength section, and a stretching component to complete the session.

• Chapter 3 deals with common problems that may arise from doing the exercises. It offers alternatives and modifications that can be used if a move proves too challenging or if you just want some variety.

• Chapter 4 covers the importance of cooling down after the cardiovascular section of the workout and gives you an easy to follow cool-down sequence.

• Chapter 5 deals with making time for relaxation and offers some relaxation techniques.

• Chapter 6 gives some guidance on how the exercises can be used to enhance sporting performance.

The CD features audio instructions for the warm-up in Chapter 1 and each of the exercises in Chapter 2, as well as the cool-down sequence in Chapter 4. The CD is intended to be a complete class to be followed from beginning to end. You can refer to the book at any time if you are not sure about a particular position.

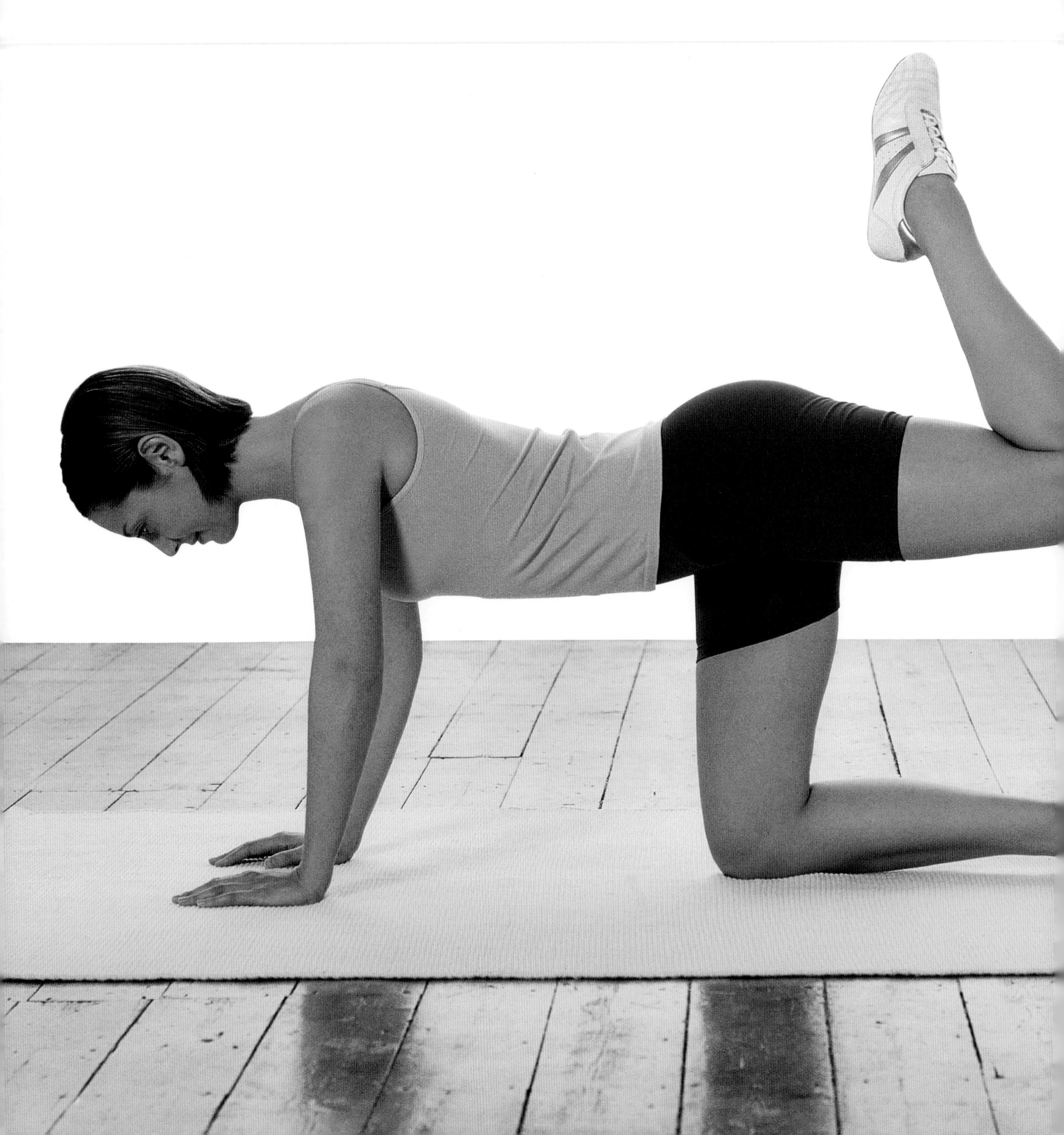

CHAPTER 1: Easy Principles

Before we start moving, I will take you through a brief outline of what fitness is. This chapter will touch on body systems and how they work so that you know why you are doing the exercises in Chapter 2. This will also increase your body awareness when doing the movements and ensure you know which muscles, joints and body systems should be working so that you can channel your effort in the right way.

We will look at the muscles that make up the core and learn how to activate these muscles to ensure stabilization as you move. I will then take you through the different elements that contribute to overall physical fitness. You will also learn how to hold yourself in a neutral posture. The workout structure is discussed and I will offer some motivational tips to help get you started and look at what you can do to keep yourself on the right track. The last section in this chapter will be the actual warm-up sequence to get you moving and on your way!

What is fitness?

The word fitness really describes a state of "being" rather than of "doing". Total fitness covers nutritional, spiritual, medical, emotional, mental, social and physical well-being. It is all about being able to live and cope well with the demands of your environment. Physical fitness, as focused on in this book, is therefore a small but crucial part of the larger picture.

The three main components of physical fitness are cardiovascular training, strength training and flexibility training. A balanced workout session will incorporate all three of these elements. These three components rely on three fundamental body systems without which we would not be able to function.

THE SKELETAL SYSTEM:

The skeletal system is the structure of bones and joints that gives the body shape. The skeleton is made so that muscles can attach at various points and movement results when the muscle contracts. The skeletal system is known as our passive system because it needs muscles to be able to move.

The skeleton also has a protective role and shields various internal organs and structures. For example: the spinal column or vertebrae protect the spinal cord; the pectoral girdle made up of ribs, collarbone, sternum and shoulder blades protects the heart and lungs; and the pelvic girdle protects the reproductive organs and the large intestine. Fitness of the skeletal system is necessary to combat bone and joint disease that will affect and restrict movement now or in the years to come.

THE MUSCULAR SYSTEM:

The muscular system is known as our active system because it is the muscle contraction that pulls on the bones to cause movement. We have to acknowledge that in the same way the skeleton needs muscle attachment and contraction to move, muscles would be useless if they had nothing to attach to.

The cardiovascular system is interrelated to the muscular system as it is the heart, lungs and blood network that supplies the muscles with the oxygen and nutrients they

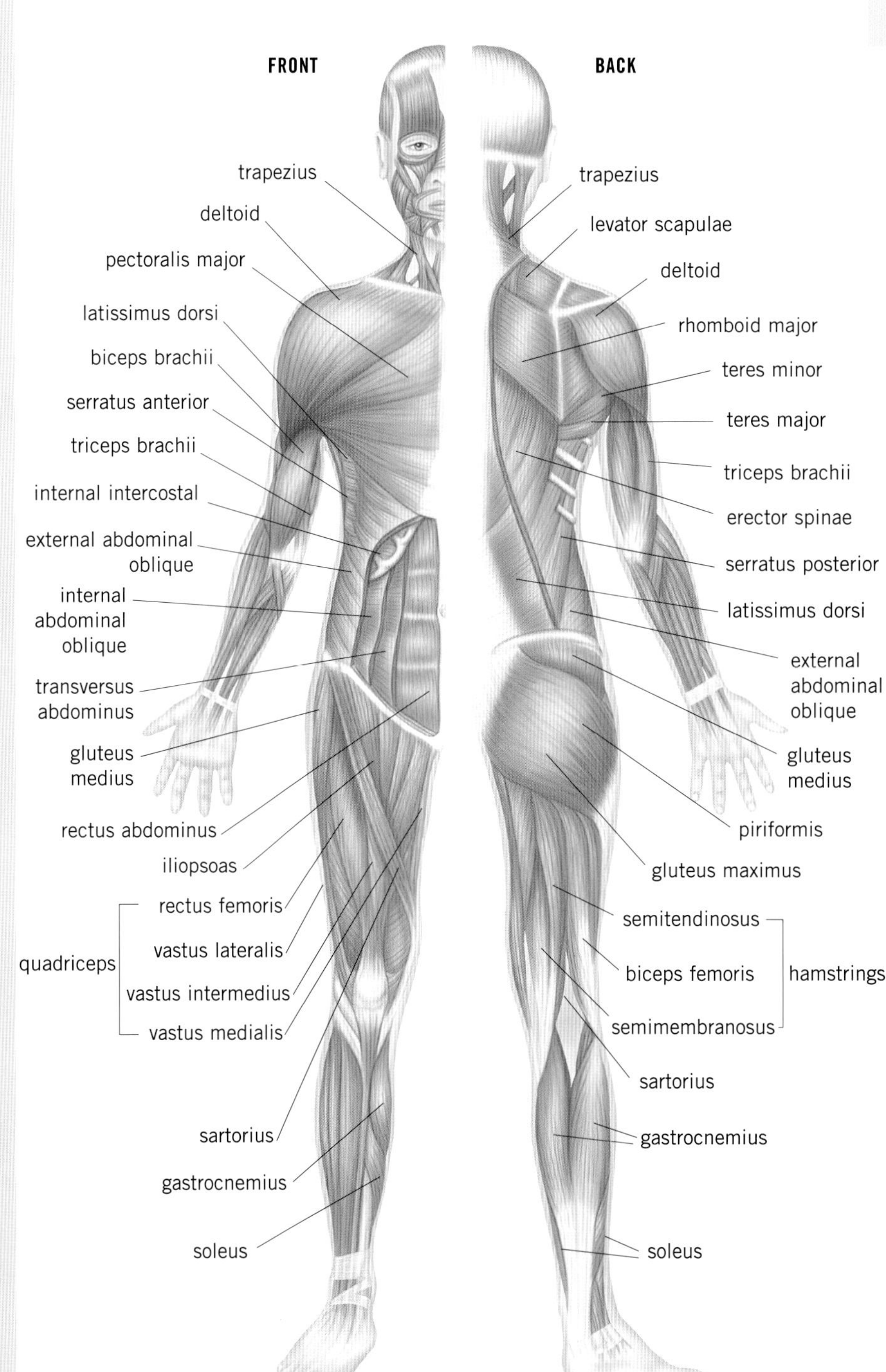

need to function effectively. The cardiovascular system also serves to carry away waste and by-products that, if left to increase beyond levels bearable by the muscle, would affect muscle function and ultimately cause a total body shut down.

Fitness of the muscular system is essential for maintaining tone and strength that reflects on movement quality and ability. Because the body can work in a variety of different positions, sometimes movements will be gravity assisted, at other times gravity is neutralized, and sometimes gravity resists the movement, making the movement harder to perform. It is important to look at muscle balance and work on any imbalances found.

Until fairly recently we essentially worked each muscle group separately. For example, we would do a bicep exercise and then a tricep exercise, followed by an exercise for the hamstrings, and then one for the gluts, etc. We would go through a list of our muscles like a shopping list. We now know from research and learning more about how the body functions that muscles should be worked in an integrated way. Many of the exercises featured in this book are combined exercises that are devised to work several muscles at once. For example, for stability, you should train the abdominals and the back together because to do so improves the working relationship they have with each other. Press-ups (see pp.56–7) are a good stabilizing exercise for working the abdominals and the back in unison.

THE NERVOUS SYSTEM:

The nervous system is probably the system we ignore the most unless we have an ache or pain. In fact, this system is known as the control system because it is the nerve impulses sent from the spinal column or the brain that cause, for example, your left leg to move. We take for granted the fact that the brain will send messages to move the left leg and the right arm forward at the same time to maintain balance in the body that prevents us from falling over to one side and ensures we move in the right direction.

We don't think about the nerve impulses that operate when we brush our teeth or eat a meal because these motor patterns that we learn at an early age have become automatic and can be done without conscious thought. We can learn new motor patterns throughout life. This is what we do when we take up rollerblading in our twenties, bowling in our forties and knitting or darts in our sixties! We also learn new motor patterns if, for example, we experience pain that makes moving difficult, or if we adopt a specific posture for long periods of time. Over time the new pattern replaces the old, so that a person may walk with a slight limp even though their ankle injury is better, or they may develop a rounded shoulder posture from sitting at a desk for long hours every day in a hunched-forward position.

Body awareness is not just about how the body is held, but also about where it is in space. Proprioreception is the ability to determine where a joint is in space. This helps the brain know if the body is off-balance. The body adapts to changes of position through sensors and receptors of the neural system. This system works joint by joint and muscle by muscle. If unchallenged, this system can get lazy and balance and coordination can suffer. Fitness of the neutral system aids the maintenance of correct and good quality movement patterns. This helps body awareness, balance and coordination and makes the sending and receiving of messages more efficient.

These systems are interdependent and integrated. If our control system is not working properly and nerve impulses are slow, reduced or non-existent because of lack of use or injury, then the muscles won't receive the impulses they require to effectively work the skeletal system and movement is limited or unable to happen.

When something goes wrong with the body it affects all systems. Take, for example, posture and alignment. Neutral alignment is good posture because "neutral" refers to the body being aligned in a way that is least stressful to the skeleton, muscles and the body's neural system. Bad posture is usually the result of muscle weakness and malfunction, muscle imbalance and a lack of body awareness. Genetic factors may pre-dispose some people toward bad posture, for example, if you are born with one leg longer than the other and you don't work on strengthening areas of concern associated with that condition. However, bad posture is usually a result of lifestyle, ways of working, sitting and standing, leisure activities, poor training programmes, etc.

The better your posture, the better you function and the lower your risk of injury. Bad posture causes a lot more stress to joints and muscles. Because bad posture often causes small stress injuries that repeatedly and frequently happen over a long period of time, aches and pains start to occur. This is a common cause of back pain.

So, what is fitness? It is about remaining healthy for daily living and developing and maintaining the ability to do any physical activity you want to try. It is about quality of life and the continuation of that quality as you get older and the body starts to deteriorate. It's about challenging the changes age brings with it and knowing that we can maintain skills, body functions and fitness levels if we work at it. We can slow down the ageing process through exercise and physical activity.

The core

The core is essentially your torso and is foundational to all movement as well as to balance, stability and coordination because it links the upper and lower body together. The condition of the core affects posture and alignment, muscle balance and muscle synergy. The core influences how you move or hold a position when you carry out your daily activities, such as carrying a bag of groceries, working at your computer, or walking around the office or home. It affects everything the body does whether it is still or moving.

The most internal part of the core is the "inner unit". Think of this unit as a can of beans. The bottom of the can is the pelvic floor muscles and the top is your diaphragm. The front and sides of the can are the deep abdominals, known as transversus abdominus. This muscle attaches into your back. The rear of the can is made up of a muscle called multifidus that runs lengthways along the spine. The beans are your internal organs! All these muscles work together to stabilize and protect the sacrum (lower spine), and the joint where the sacrum and pelvis meet.

Stabilization happens when the pelvic floor, deep abdominals and back muscles are simultaneously switched on. To activate your pelvic floor, imagine you want to stop yourself urinating or that you want to get into a pair of jeans that are a half size too small. Your pelvic floor muscles will contract and tighten. Keep the activation and pull your navel toward your spine. Try to maintain the natural curve in your lower back. Your waist should feel smaller and firmer. If you are holding your breath, you have drawn in too much. Breathe normally.

The muscles of the bottom and hips, upper back and legs, and the other abdominals and lower back make up the "outer unit" of the core, which also contributes to stabilization.

First you need to train your body to keep the inner core muscles activated for longer periods of time. Second, you should practise maintaining this as you move. Third, you want to be able to activate these muscles automatically, so that you can maintain stabilization without thinking about it.

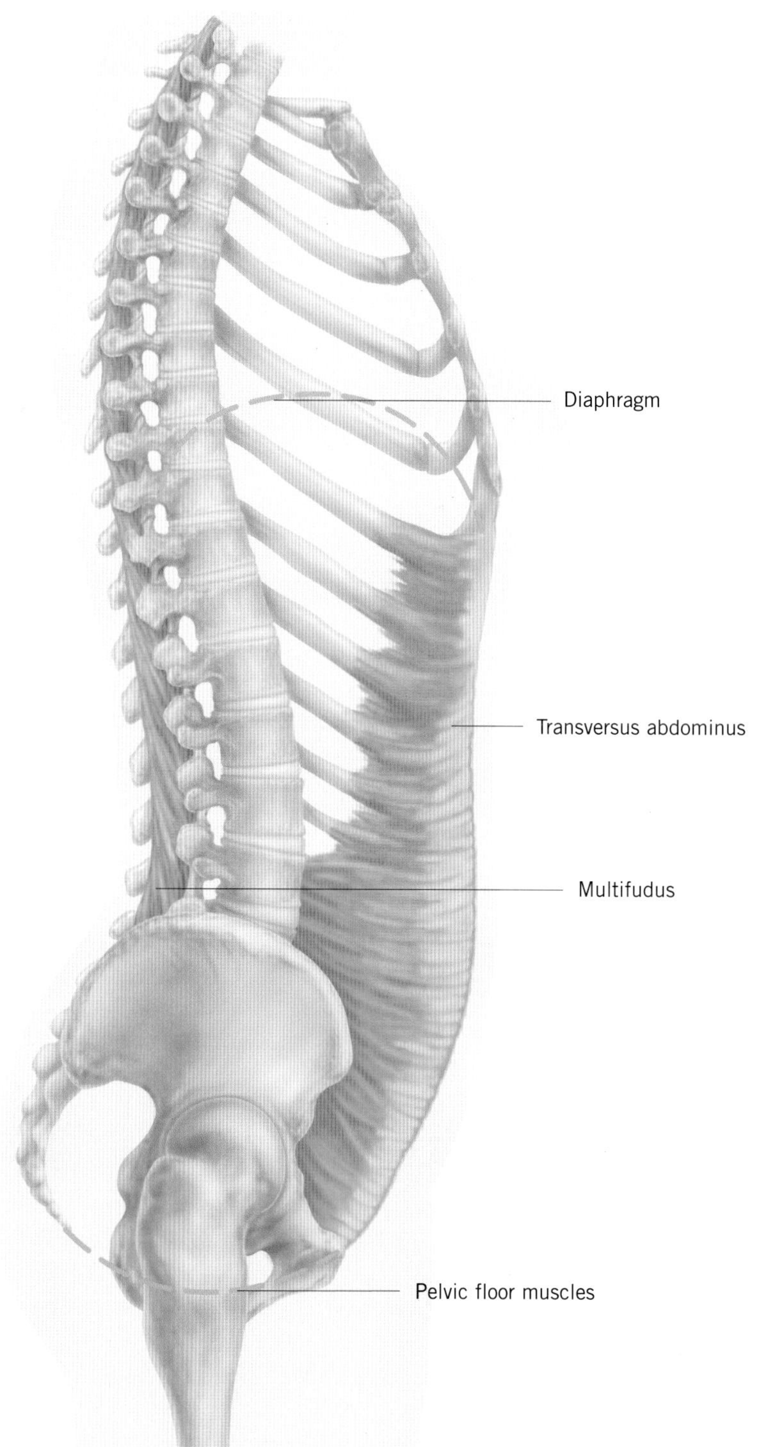

The six elements of fitness

A well-rounded and complete fitness session will have six sections: it begins with a warm-up, followed by cardiovascular training and then a cool-down. Next there is a strengthening section and a flexibility section. A relaxation session concludes the workout. Sometimes these sections are quite distinct and sometimes, depending on what movements you do and how you do them, parts of your workout can be combined or serve more than one purpose. All of the exercises and stretches in your *Easy Fitness Workbook* have been chosen because they are integrated (work the upper and lower body together) and compound (work across more than one joint), so that they can be time efficient as well as functional.

THE WARM-UP:

The warm-up is a vital starting point for any session or activity. This is when the body gently and progressively gets prepared for the work that is to come. The objective is to take the body from a resting state to an active state with the least amount of stress and discomfort, and so the activity should not be a shock for the body.

The warm-up and the cool-down are essentially the beginning and the end of the cardiovascular section. The movements done in the warm-up section will usually mimic what is to be done in the main segment, so that it acts as a physical and mental rehearsal. By the time you finish the warm-up, you should be psychologically and physically ready for the main section of the workout.

The warm-up has different components. There should be some mobility exercises to prepare the joints. These exercises warm up the synovial fluid within the joint capsule. This aids joint lubrication and results in easier and greater range of movement, and less risk of injury and soreness.

The mobility exercises may be separate from or combined with large, rhythmical movements involving the bigger muscles of the lower body. These rhythmical movements increase heart and breathing rate so that the cardiovascular system, including the lungs, gets prepared to pump more blood and oxygen around the body. Body temperature will rise and muscles get warmer and more pliable as a result. Think of a car that might stutter and jerk a little when it's cold and first gets started, but runs more smoothly as it gets warmed up.

The warm-up also causes an increase in neural impulses. This accelerates the process of transmitting messages between the brain, the spine and the muscles. In addition, the psychological aspect of the warm-up contributes to a heightened sense of body awareness that improves performance ability.

The warm-up may include a pre-workout stretch to help prepare the muscles for activity. Some research suggests that doing a pre-workout stretch may also decrease the risk of muscular or joint injury.

CARDIOVASCULAR SECTION:

The cardiovascular section is included to train the heart and lungs and to improve the efficiency of the circulatory system. Cardiovascular fitness is sometimes referred to as cardiovascular endurance or stamina. It dictates how long someone will be able to work at a particular level of intensity before they get fatigued and have to stop. When the cardiovascular (otherwise known as the cardiorespiratory) system is stressed by activity, the system adapts and becomes better at dealing with the new levels of intensity. It becomes more efficient at taking in oxygen, transporting it in the blood and extracting it when it gets to the muscles. The body also gets better at using the oxygen to produce aerobic energy once the oxygen reaches the cells of the muscle. The heart adapts by pumping more blood for the same amount of effort, or with less effort.

COOL-DOWN:

The cool-down is as important as the warm-up. The main cool-down should be done immediately after the cardiovascular segment. The objective is to gradually return the body to its pre-exercise, resting state. The movements go from large to small, intense to less intense, to gradually bring down the heart rate, temperature and breathing rate.

The cool-down also allows the circulatory system to reduce blood flow to the muscles and divert some of that blood back to other systems and organs, such as the digestive system. After the cardiovascular section, a lot of the body's blood supply will be in the legs. Actively cooling down simply means you keep moving, and so aid blood return to the heart and brain and prevent blood pooling in the legs.

STRENGTHENING SECTION:

There are two sub-components to resistance training: strength of the muscles and endurance. Strength relates to how much weight you can lift or move while endurance focuses on how long you can continuously lift or move a weight before fatigue sets in.

At base level we should all be able to lift or move our own body weight to get out of a chair or walk a distance. For some people this is a struggle and a definite sign that they are not as healthy as they could be. If you fall into this category, find resistance training particularly problematic or it is new to you, you should start by working and training to be active with your own body weight before adding external weight, such as dumb-bells, ankle weights and weighted bars.

Both strength and endurance add tone to muscle, but strength will involve a greater increase in muscle size and probably more definition. Women often shy away from doing "heavy" weights for fear of becoming too muscular and looking like a body builder. However, in reality, because of the difference in male and female hormones, a female who trains with heavier weights should retain her female body shape and would only end up looking like a male body builder if drugs, such as steroids, were taken.

FLEXIBILITY SECTION:

The words "flexibility" and "stretching" are often used interchangeably to mean the same thing, but flexibility is the desired state and stretching is how you get there.

There are "normal" degrees of range of motion that can be used to measure flexibility. For example, your hamstrings should be flexible enough so that if you lie on your back, you should be able to lift your leg and flex at your hip to 90 degrees. If you cannot do this, your hamstrings probably need stretching (unless the limitation in movement is caused by muscle bulk, body mass or injury). However, If you exceed 90 degrees and can get your ankle to your ear, you may be too flexible. Excessively flexible or hypermobile joints can be more easily dislocated if there is insufficient muscle tone to stabilize the joint. People that are hypermobile need to be careful not to overstretch.

All muscles, from the neck down, should be stretched at some time during your week's workouts. You can also have a stretch session (this could be yoga based, but it doesn't have to be) to specifically address flexibility or your flexibility section can be part of your final cool-down and used to relax certain muscles, especially if you don't have time for a dedicated relaxation segment.

Remember that stretches can be done for maintenance of existing levels of flexibility or to develop flexibility. Maintenance stretches are usually held for 8–10 seconds, whereas developmental stretches are held for at least 30 seconds. With a developmental stretch you are waiting for the release of tension and tightness in the muscle. This is the signal for you to ease a little bit further into the stretch to try to lengthen beyond the original state.

RELAXATION SECTION:

This component of a session has great benefits for the mind and the body and yet it is often skipped. Try to make time for relaxation. Treat it as reward for having done all the hard work!

You can totally relax and let go, emptying your mind of all preoccupying thoughts, or you can guide your thoughts while focusing on your breathing. Use this time to release any residual tension if you are going to be restful afterwards or to re-energize if you have to get up and be active.

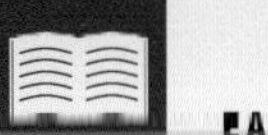

Neutral alignment

Before you start any exercise or movement, you should consider neutral posture relative to the exercise position, unless the exercise instructions specify otherwise.

To position yourself in a neutral standing posture, do the following awareness exercise.

- Stand with your feet hip-distance apart, parallel and facing forward.
- Ensure your weight is evenly distributed through the whole area of each foot.
- Your knees and hips should be over your ankles and facing the same direction.
- Your knees should be very slightly bent.
- Your pelvis should be level, right to left and centred so that your tailbone points downward.
- Your core muscles must be switched on before you move and tone held in these muscles throughout the movement.
- Your spine needs to be long with a natural concave curve in your lower back and neck.
- Your chest should be open with your shoulders rolled back and your shoulder blades pulling down your back. Check that your ribs are not flaring – they should be eased down, close to your abdominals.
- Your arms should fall alongside the body with your palms facing in toward the side of your thighs and your thumbs facing forward.
- Hold your neck long, with its natural curve.
- Your head should sit centrally on your shoulders with your chin drawn in toward the base of your skull.

• The crown of your head should be easing up toward the ceiling.

• If you stand alongside a straight, vertical line, eg the edge of a door or door frame, the line should pass through your earlobe and shoulder joint, just behind your hip joint and just in front of your knee and ankle joints.

If you find it hard to stand as directed you may have a posture type that is not neutral. This will be evident in the position of your pelvis and tailbone or the rounding of your shoulders and closing in of your chest. You may be lordotic, where the pelvis is tilted forward, exaggerating the curve in the lower back; kyphotic, where the shoulders roll in and the chest contracts, exaggerating the curve in the upper back; swayback, where the hip joint moves forward of the posture line; or flatback, where the curve in the lower back is reduced.

Work on trying to achieve the neutral posture position by stretching whatever feels tight and is shortened, relaxing whatever feels tight but has a good length and strengthening whatever is weak and over-lengthened.

Even when you change from a standing position to seated or lying position, you should run through this checklist. If your knees are bent and your feet are on the floor, you should still have a small curve in your lower back. If your knees are bent and your feet are off the floor, you could lightly press your lower back into the floor to help support your spine.

Creating a fitness regime

Starting a new regime can be daunting. There may be certain barriers that you have to overcome before you can start exercising.

Some people create a barrier for themselves when they equate exercise with "being sporty" and they don't see themselves as a sporty person. Self-perception dictates how we see ourselves and what we do or don't do as a consequence. Acknowledge that you don't have to view yourself as sporty to do this workout and that the workout is aimed at improving health and general fitness rather than sporting performance.

Another barrier may be caused by past experiences of exercise. For example, at school you may have been made to do activities you did not enjoy. Those negative memories and feelings can carry over to the present day. You need to overcome those feelings by recognizing that this is a different situation and that you are in control; you can choose to do activities you enjoy or learn new ones and you can stop at any time and try something different.

A training buddy is a good idea to get you started and keep you motivated, but you must be committed to still doing the activity even if they have to skip a session!

It often helps if you have specific goals or objectives for your training. You could set yourself the task of walking a certain distance or improving your time over a set distance.

You could aim to take part in a small race event to raise money for charity. Your goals can be anything from swimming a certain number of lengths in a set time, to taking part in a rollerblading event or doing a skydive!

Remember to make "smart" goals. They should be specific, measurable, achievable, recorded and have a time frame. If you have set yourself a big goal, focusing on the little steps toward that goal, for example, the commitment to work out three times per week and what you are going to do in those three sessions, is more important than focusing on the big goal because if you carry out the little steps you will achieve the bigger goal. If you focus on the bigger goal without a clear idea of what to do to achieve it, you can get lost and demotivated.

Schedule when you are going to work out. We are often more committed to things when we write them down. If you really can't make a session, don't beat yourself up, just reschedule! This also acts as a record. You can go back and see how many times you have worked out for the month. Give yourself a pat on the back when you achieve most of what you intended. Better still, have a reward system. This could be a meal at your favourite restaurant, a facial or a massage, buying a new gadget or, to mark the bigger achievements, something more extravagant, like a spa day, a weekend away or a holiday.

Easy workout warm-up

The key objective in doing a warm-up is to make the exercise experience effective and safe and the transition from not exercising to exercising smooth and comfortable.

Pre-workout stretches may be included toward the end of the warm-up, once the muscles are warm. These are used to lengthen the muscles that may be tight from daily postures and activities. If someone has been sitting or in a static posture all day, they can ease muscles out before getting them to work. The pre-workout stretches will generally involve static (holding) stretches held for 8 to 10 seconds. The problem with this is that the body may start cooling down as the stretches are held. However, the stretch positions can actually be held actively (where other muscles have to work to hold the stretch position) instead of passively (where the muscles relax into the stretch and are not really working). Because some muscles have to work during active stretching, the body is kept warmer.

If a pre-stretch is not done, the muscles should be taken through dynamic, full range movement in a slow and controlled manner to lengthen the muscle while it moves. This can be done as part of the rhythmical movements. Dynamic movements for the hamstrings, calves and quadriceps have been included in this warm-up sequence. You might want to do some static stretching for these muscles and for the shoulders and hip flexors if they feel tight.

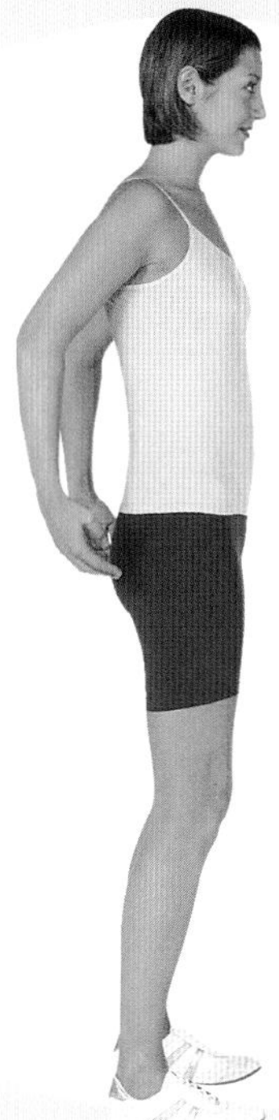

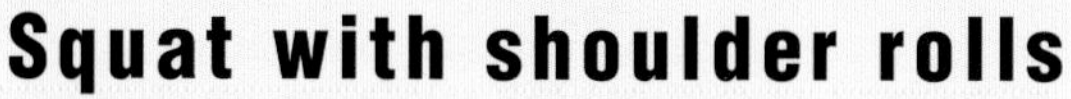

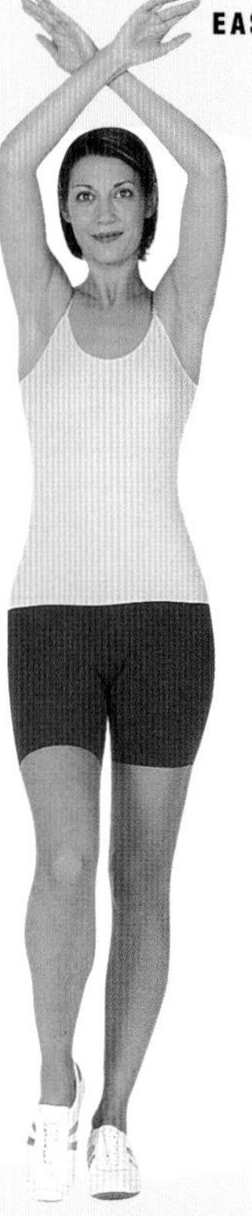

Squat with shoulder rolls

Stand in neutral with you feet hip-distance apart. Bend at your hips and knees and sit back, as if you were going to sit on a chair. Squeeze your gluteals (bottom muscles) as you straighten yourself up and stand tall. Combine a shoulder roll with the squat. Your shoulders should move forward of the body and lift toward your ears as you sit back. Take them behind your body and press them away from your ears as you stand up. Repeat 20 times.

March with arm circles

March on the spot at a moderate pace. Bend your elbows and pump your arms forward and back, as if you were marching on parade. Exaggerate your arms. Once you have done this for a minute, keep marching and circle your arms in front of you. Take your arms out to the side, lift them above your head and cross them as you bring them down in front of your body. Repeat 16 times, then circle your arms the other way for 16 repetitions.

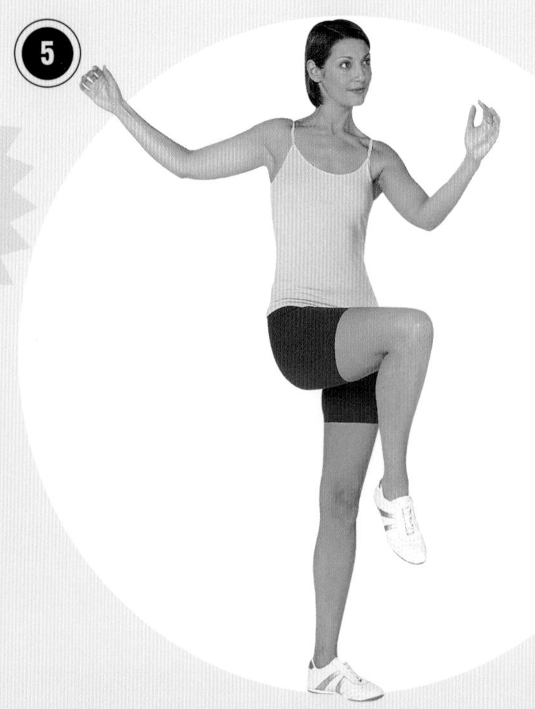
5

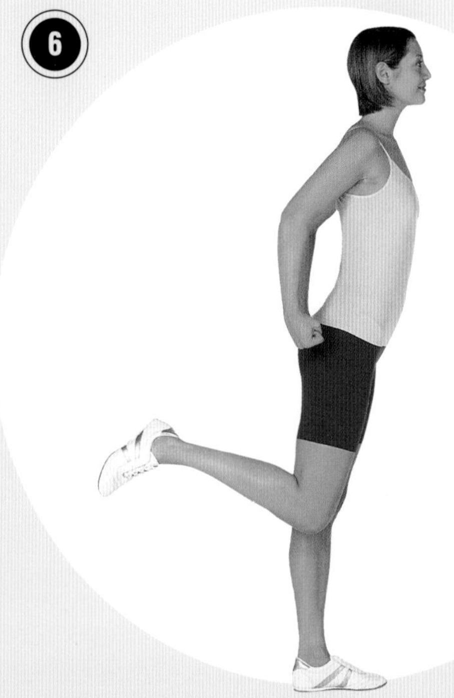
6

Knee lift with opposite elbow to knee

Stand tall and in neutral. Lift your right knee so that it is about level with your hip and cross your left elbow over toward your right knee. Maintain a long spine and make sure you are not leaning forward. Aim to take your knee toward your chest rather than your chest toward your knee. Replace your right leg. Lift your left leg and bring your right elbow across. Repeat this sequence 20 times.

Hamstring curls with tricep kickbacks

Stand in neutral with your feet a little more than hip-distance apart. Bend your elbows and pull your arms behind you. Bend your right knee and lift your heel toward your bottom. Replace your right leg and do the same with your left. As your legs are raised and replaced, your arms should straighten and bend. Keep your elbows in the same place as you move your arms. Repeat this sequence 20 times.

7

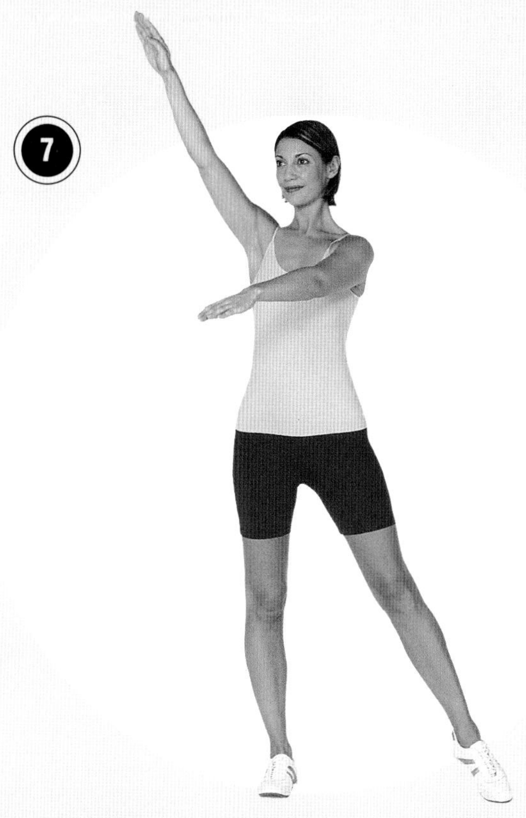

8

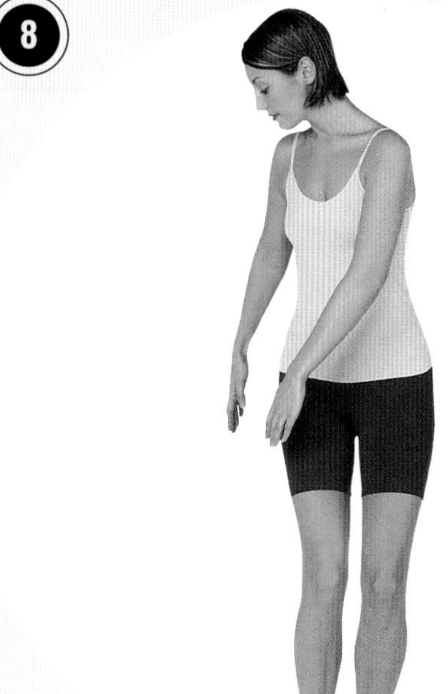

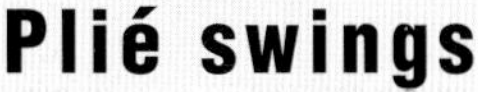

Plié swings

A plié is a type of wide squat, where, rather than bending forward from the hips, the back remains upright. Take a wide stance with your feet slightly turned out. Check that your knees and feet face the same direction. Sit into the position, lowering your hips toward the level of your knees. Keep your back upright. Stand up and swing your arms to your right. Plié again, bringing your arms low in front of you. Swing to the left. Repeat 20 times on each side.

Heel raise with cross chop

Stand with your feet hip-distance apart, looking straight ahead. Lift up onto your toes and take your arms up toward the left side of your head. Look toward your hands. As you lower your heels, take your arms across your body so that your hands are by the outside of your right thigh. Bend your knees a little. Remember to look in the direction of your hands. Repeat 20 times on one side and then change over and repeat 20 times on the other side.

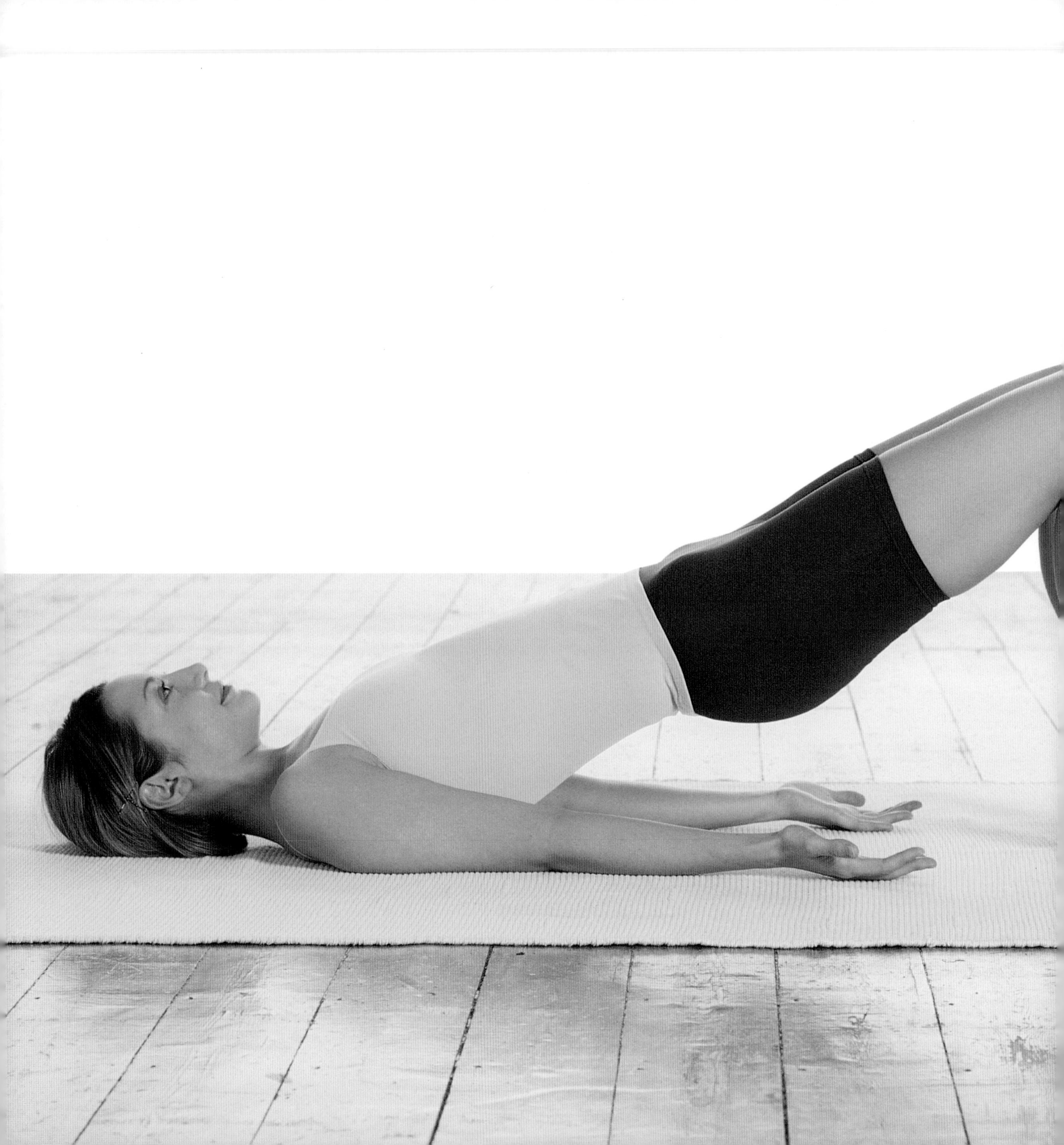

CHAPTER 2: Easy Workout

The 20 exercises included in this section cover the cardiovascular, strength and flexibility components of a workout. This combination of activities will challenge the three body systems – the muscular, the skeletal and the nervous systems – working all three simultaneously is essential when fitness for daily function is a high priority. Modern fitness training is moving away from isolating specific muscle groups and working each one separately, as this approach does not reflect how the body operates in real life. Although we may occasionally focus more on one aspect than on another, all of the exercises require a mixture of strength and flexibility and work a number of different joints and muscles at the same time. You will need an exercise mat (or a thick towel), a chair without arms and a sturdy stool (if you don't have stairs). You will also be using parts of your home such as a wall, floorspace and the stairs.

Step-ups with chest press

GOOD FOR: working all the muscles of the lower body at the same time

TAKE CARE IF: you suffer from mild knee problems. Use something no higher than a normal stair

AVOID IF: you suffer from severe knee problems

SEE P.80

Find a step, some stairs, or something that you can safely step up and down on, such as a low, sturdy stool. Start with your arms at chest level with your elbows pointing back. Step up with your right foot and press your arms out in front of you. Then step up with your left foot and pull your arms back to the start position. Step down with your right foot and then your left foot, repeating the same arm action. Repeat this movement for 45 seconds. Change legs, so that you step up and down with your left foot first. Repeat for another 45 seconds.

NOTES

The action of stepping up and down helps to tone, strengthen and increase the muscular endurance of all the major leg muscles. At the same time, the inner and outer thigh muscles and the muscles around the pelvis need to work to stabilize the knee joints and pelvis. Inclusion of the arms helps to tone the arms and chest and works on stabilizing the back muscles.

Adopt a neutral posture before and during the exercise. This will improve posture and alignment. Ensure that you place your whole foot on the step. This helps to distribute the impact through the whole foot rather than just one section (eg the ball of your foot) and ensures that your body weight is evenly dispersed and that you are properly balanced on the step.

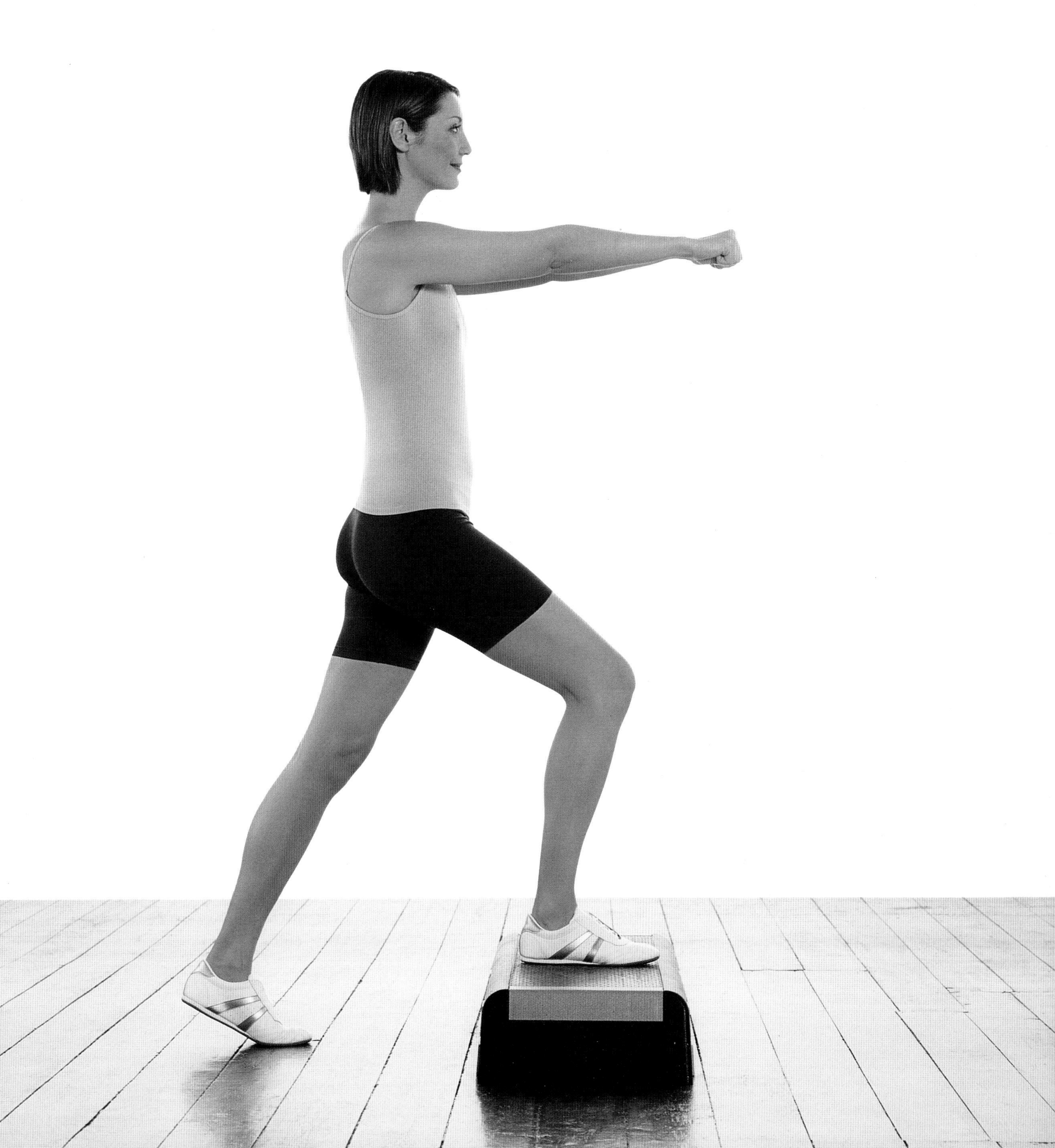

Sprint-runs

GOOD FOR: working on agility, speed and general mobility

TAKE CARE IF: you have knee or ankle joint problems. Decrease the speed – you will still benefit if you do the exercise at a gentle jogging pace

SEE P.81

Clear some space in a room, corridor or garden. If the space is long enough you can run from one end to the other. If it is a small space, set out some markers at 2–3 feet (60cm–1 metre) intervals. Run from your start point to the first marker and back to the start point. Then run to the second marker and back to the start point. Continue like this for each of your markers and then repeat the whole series. You should perform the sprint-runs for 90 seconds.

NOTES

This exercise targets the muscles of the legs as well as muscles around the shoulder joint. While some muscles are causing the arm to move others hold the shoulder joint in a strong position as the movement takes place. Although the sprint-run action primarily happens in the lower body, the arms contribute to coordination as they move to counterbalance the movement of the lower body. Switching on your core muscles before you move helps keep your torso strong while your limbs are executing the movements.

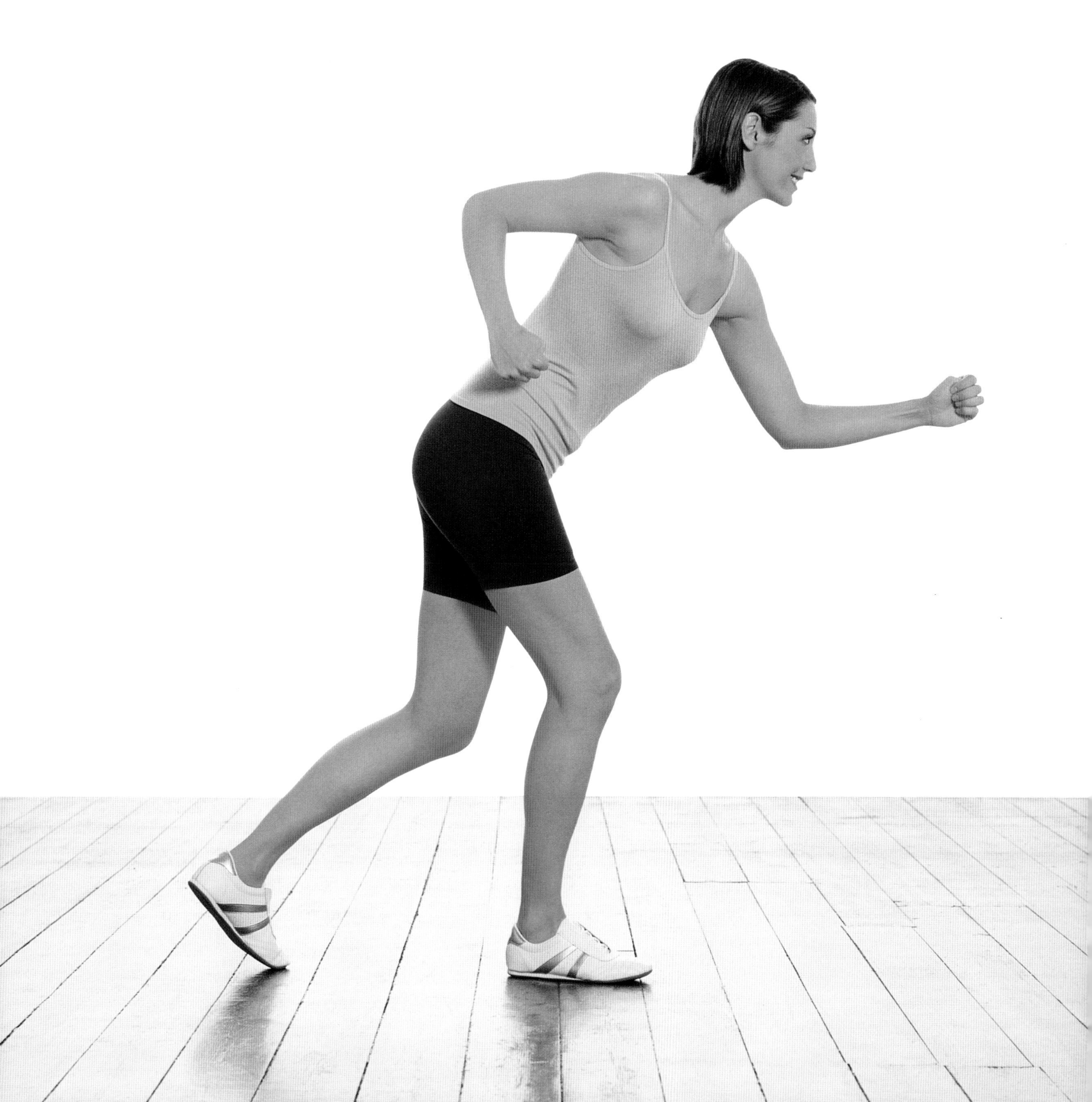

Jumping twists

11

GOOD FOR: strengthening the oblique abdominal muscles. Provides controlled impact that can help prevent or reduce the risk of osteoporosis

TAKE CARE IF: you already suffer from osteoporosis

SEE P.82

Stand with your feet and legs together. Bend your knees slightly. Activate your pelvic floor, deep abdominals and back muscles. Jump on the spot and use your arms to help twist your upper body in one direction while your lower body twists in the opposite direction. The power of the twist and the jump should come from the torso, rather than just the legs. Repeat for 90 seconds, as vigorously as possible. As you jump, remember to alternate the direction of your twists.

NOTES

The twisting action involves the external and internal oblique abdominals, transversus abdominus and the other elements of the core. The jumping action works the major hip and thigh muscles as well as the muscles of the lower leg. This activity helps to tone, strengthen and increase the muscular endurance and power of the legs. The inner thigh muscles work as stabilizers as they help keep the thighs and knees together. The stabilizing muscles of the pelvis are also working to hold the pelvis level and stop it tilting from side to side. Stabilization of the back is essential to ensure that the arms move freely but with control so that there is no risk to the back (eg pulling a muscle).

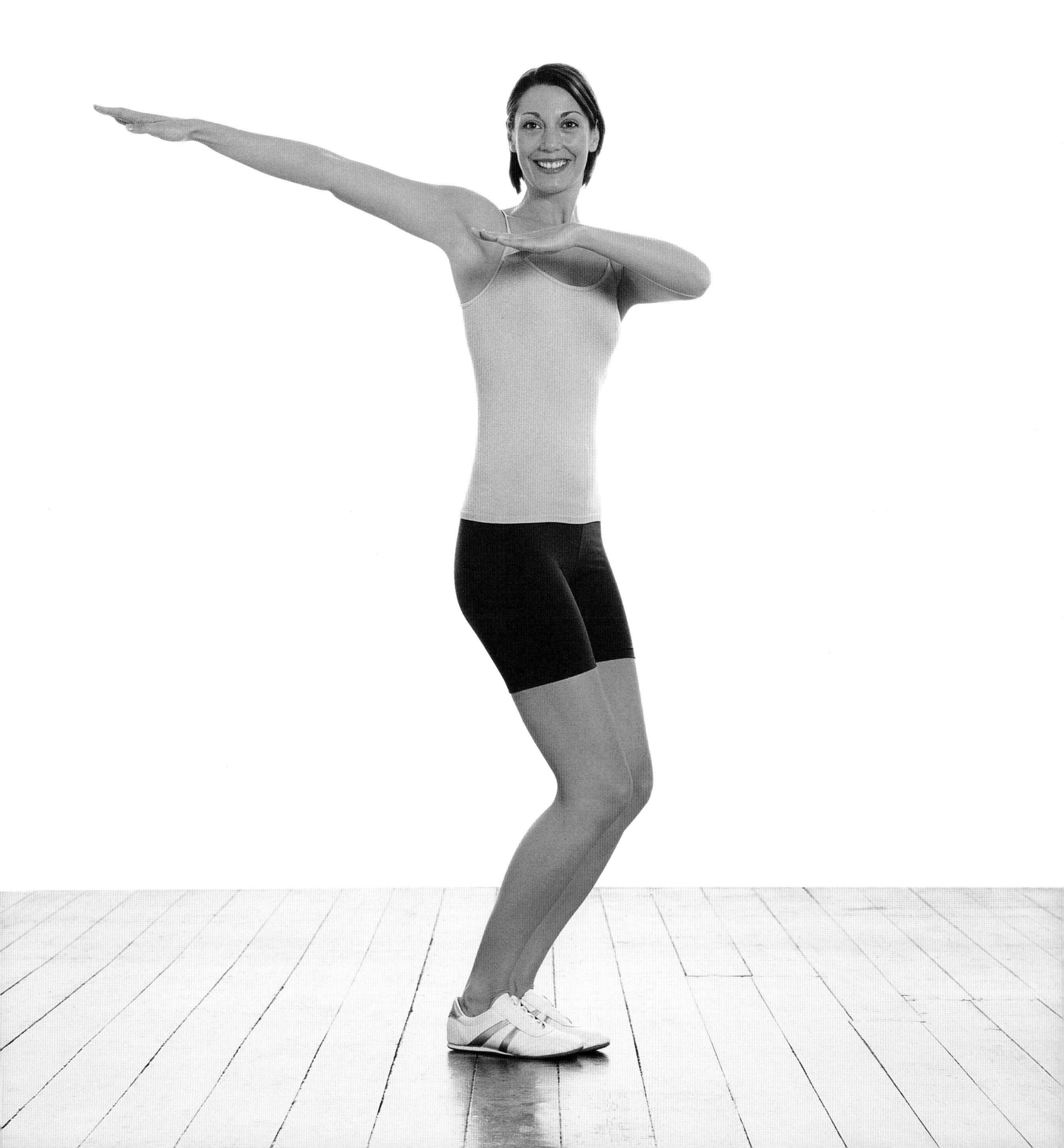

Knee lifts with arms overhead

GOOD FOR: focusing on posture; overall workout

TAKE CARE IF: you suffer from mild knee problems. Use something no higher than a stair

AVOID IF: you suffer from severe knee problems

SEE P.83

Stand in front of the step or stair with your arms by your side. Step up with your right foot and bend your elbows, bringing your hands level with your shoulders, as if you were doing a bicep curl. While you balance on your right leg, lift your left knee to hip level and push your arms above your head. Replace your left foot on the floor, bringing your hands back to shoulder level. Step down with your right foot, replacing your arms by your side. Then change legs. Repeat for 90 seconds, remembering to alternate legs.

NOTES

This exercise tones, strengthens and increases the muscular endurance of the legs and hips. The inner and outer thigh muscles work to stabilize the knee joints. The muscles at the side of the hip work to hold the pelvis in position so that it does not tilt from side to side or forward or backward. This in turn keeps the spine in neutral and helps to maintain good posture and alignment. The arm action works to tone and strengthen the muscles of the shoulder and improve their endurance. The back muscles are involved as stabilizers. Making sure that you place your whole foot on the step is as crucial here as it is in the Step-ups (see p.36), for the same reasons. Good balance and proper alignment is even more important when standing on one leg.

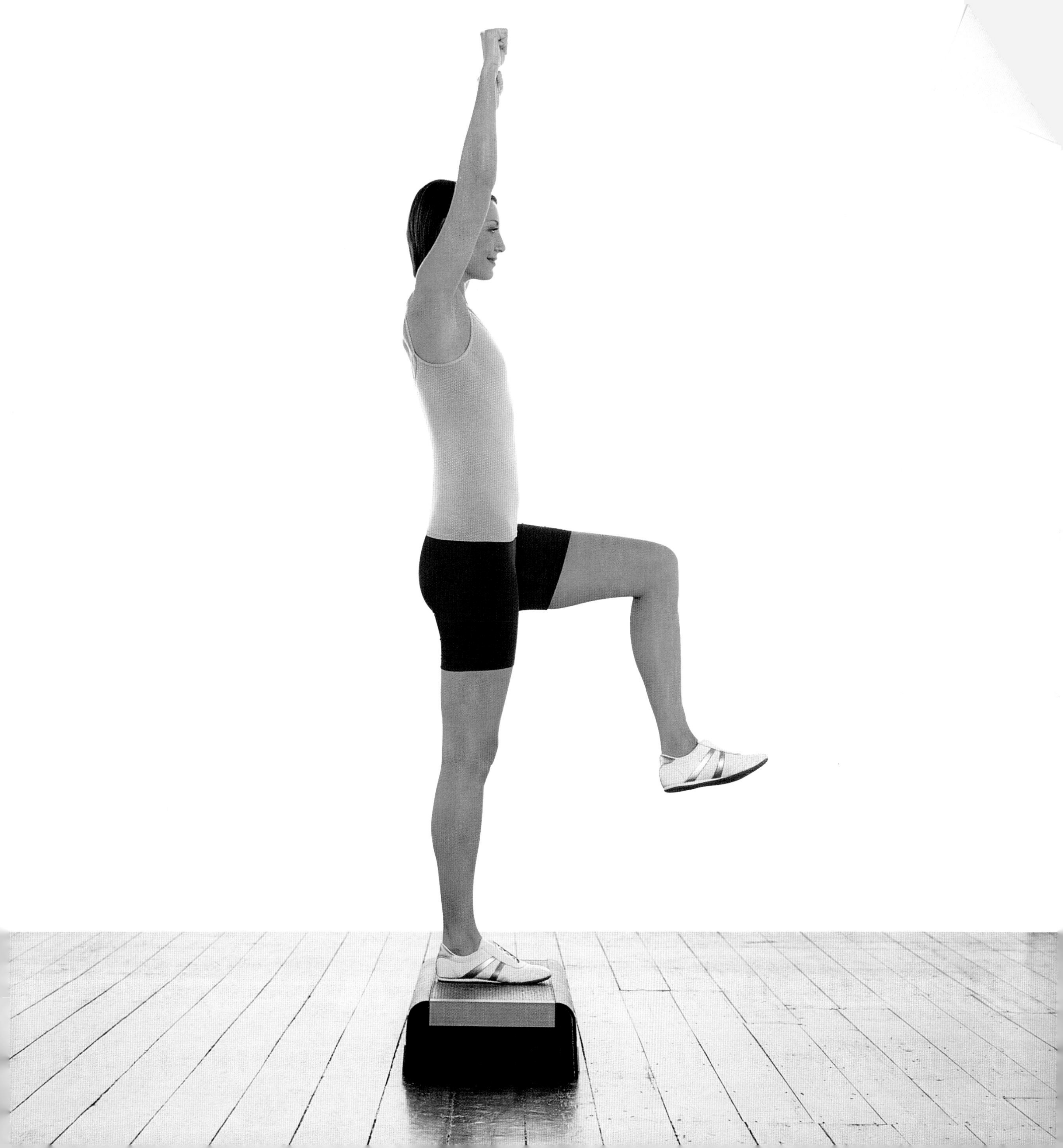

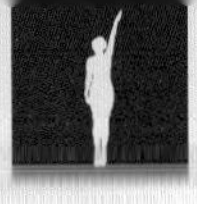

Wall jumps

13

GOOD FOR: sports such as basketball or netball

TAKE CARE IF: you have knee or ankle joint problems

AVOID IF: you suffer from: disc problems or bone problems such as osteoporosis

SEE P.84

Make an imaginary mark high up on a wall about 2–3 feet (60cm–1 metre) above where your hand reaches if you stand by the wall and reach up with your arm. Walk back 3 feet (1 metre). This is your start position. Run forward and jump to touch the mark. Shuffle back to the start position. Repeat this exercise for 45 seconds, trying to jump as high as you can. Now stand where you have been jumping, turn yourself around and run to what was your start position, jump and reach with your other arm. Then shuffle back. Repeat for 45 seconds.

NOTES

This exercise works the legs quite explosively and improves endurance levels specifically in the legs as well as the heart and lungs. The inner and outer thighs stabilize the knees. The core muscles should be activated to hold the torso strong and safe as you prepare and then execute the jumps. Ensure you bend your knees before you jump and on landing.

The core (inner unit), back and shoulder muscles will also be involved as you bend forward to prepare to jump and then lift your body up and extend your torso and arm to touch the mark. Swing your arms back before you jump to help with the upward lift.

Here, the body is trained as a "whole unit", where every muscle is doing something.

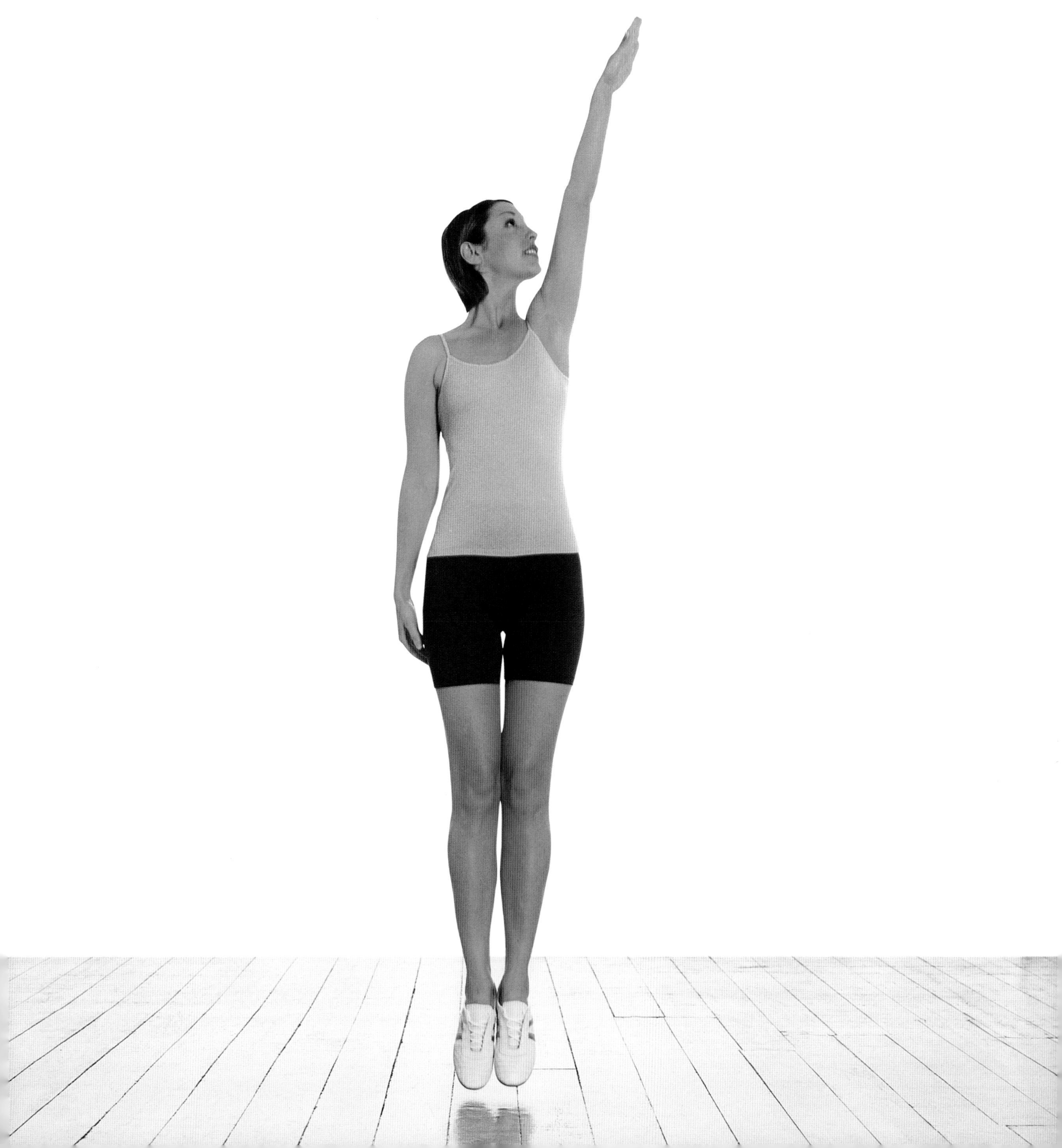

Line skiing

14

GOOD FOR:
skiing preparation: leg strength and endurance

TAKE CARE IF:
you have knee or ankle joint problems

AVOID IF:
you suffer from disc problems or bone problems such as osteoporosis

SEE P.85

Find a line on your carpet, tiled or wooden floor, or make a line with some string, tape, etc. Stand on one side of the line with your feet together. Switch on your core muscles. Bend your knees and jump side to side across the line in a ski action. With your elbows bent, push your arms forward as you take off and pull your elbows behind you as you land on the other side of the line. Try to look forward rather than down at the floor as you jump. Perform this exercise for 90 seconds.

NOTES

The legs are a key component of this exercise and the muscles of the hip and pelvis should be working to stabilize. Activating core muscles first will keep the body safe as the lift and landing occur. Many people translate the skiing action as one that causes the pelvis to tilt from side to side. In fact, the pelvis should stay level as the whole body shifts over the line. This reduces the stress placed on the joints, especially the knees and ankles and the lateral stress through the spine. Keeping your eyes forward ensures good head and neck position and better upper body posture. The arm movement assists the lift and emphasizes the fact that the upper and lower body will always naturally counterbalance each other.

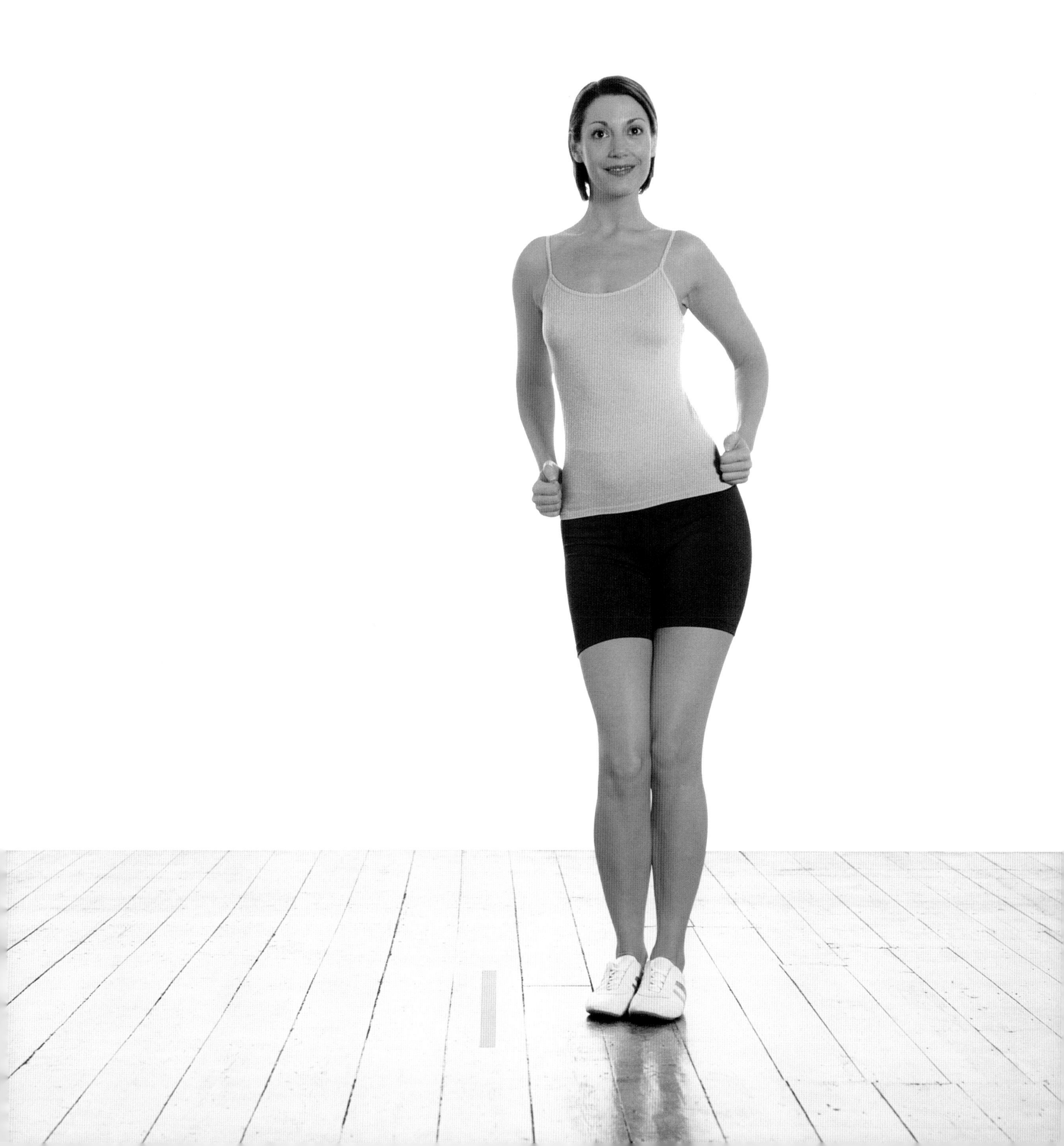

Single leg squats

19

GOOD FOR: working lots of muscles at the same time; developing balance skills

TAKE CARE IF: you have hip, knee and/or ankle problems or balance issues

SEE PP.86–7

Stand with your feet hip-distance apart and with your spine and pelvis in neutral. Engage your core muscles. Lift one foot off the floor and straighten it out in front of you. Bend at your hips and squat back, as if you were going to sit down. As you squat, keep your lifted leg in front of you (with your toes pointed) and push your arms forward, lifting them to chest level. Take your arms back down by your side as you stand up. Take 4 counts to lower your hips and 4 counts to return to standing. Start with whatever number of repetitions you can do with good technique and balance, and work up to 16 repetitions on each leg.

NOTES

This is a very efficient and effective total body exercise that strengthens both the front and rear thigh and buttock muscles. Focus on using your inner and outer thigh muscles to stabilize the knee as it bends and straightens as this will improve the integrity of the knee joint. Ensure your core muscles are activated to hold your spine in neutral. Your pelvis and shoulder blades also need to be stabilized so that they hold and maintain position as you move. Ensure that the forward bend happens at the hip joint and not through the spine. Keep your chest open and your shoulder blades sliding down toward your waist.

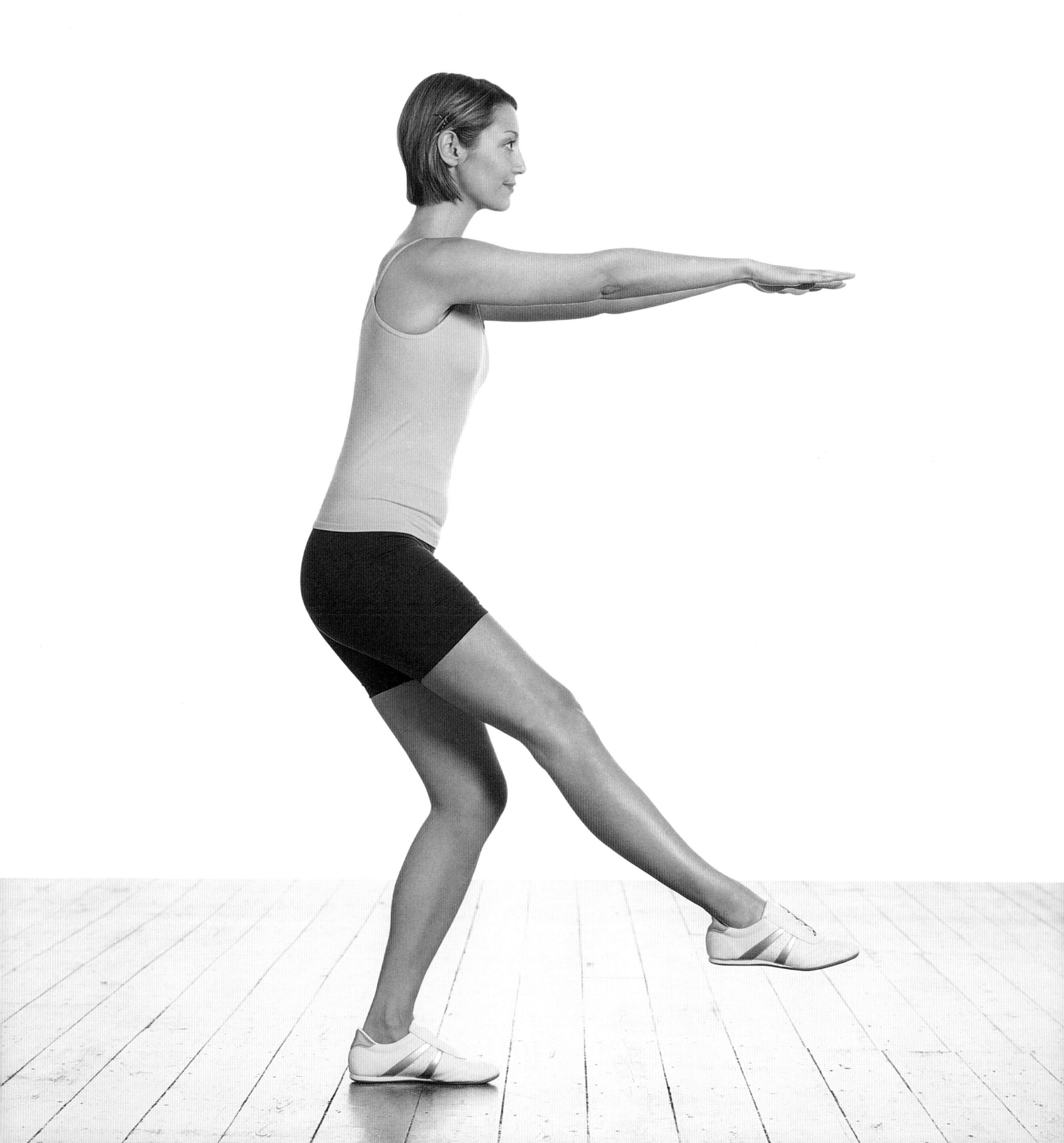

Lunge, knee lift and cross chop

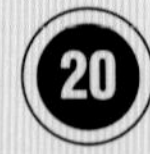

GOOD FOR: strengthening the legs for day to day function, eg walking; balance; shoulder stabilization

TAKE CARE IF: you have balance issues; knee or ankle joint problems

SEE PP.88–9

Start with your feet hip-distance apart and step your right foot behind you, keeping your heel lifted. Bend your right knee toward the floor as you lunge, keeping your knee in line with your hip joint. Place both hands by your right hip. Simultaneously take your arms above your head to the left side in a chopping action and lift your right knee up to hip height. As you replace your foot behind you, take your arms across your body and down to your right hip. Take 2 seconds to lift your knee and 2 seconds to take your foot back. Do 16 repetitions on each side.

NOTES

The quadriceps, hamstrings, gluteals and hip flexors are at work in this movement. The inner and outer thighs are involved to stabilize the knees, and the pelvis must stay level and aligned with the spine. Ensure your front knee remains above and in line with your ankle and does not push over your toes. Check that your hips face forward and don't tilt to either side when you are in the lunge position or when you lift your knee. When lifting your arms, try to keep your shoulders and shoulder blades pressed down, away from your ears.

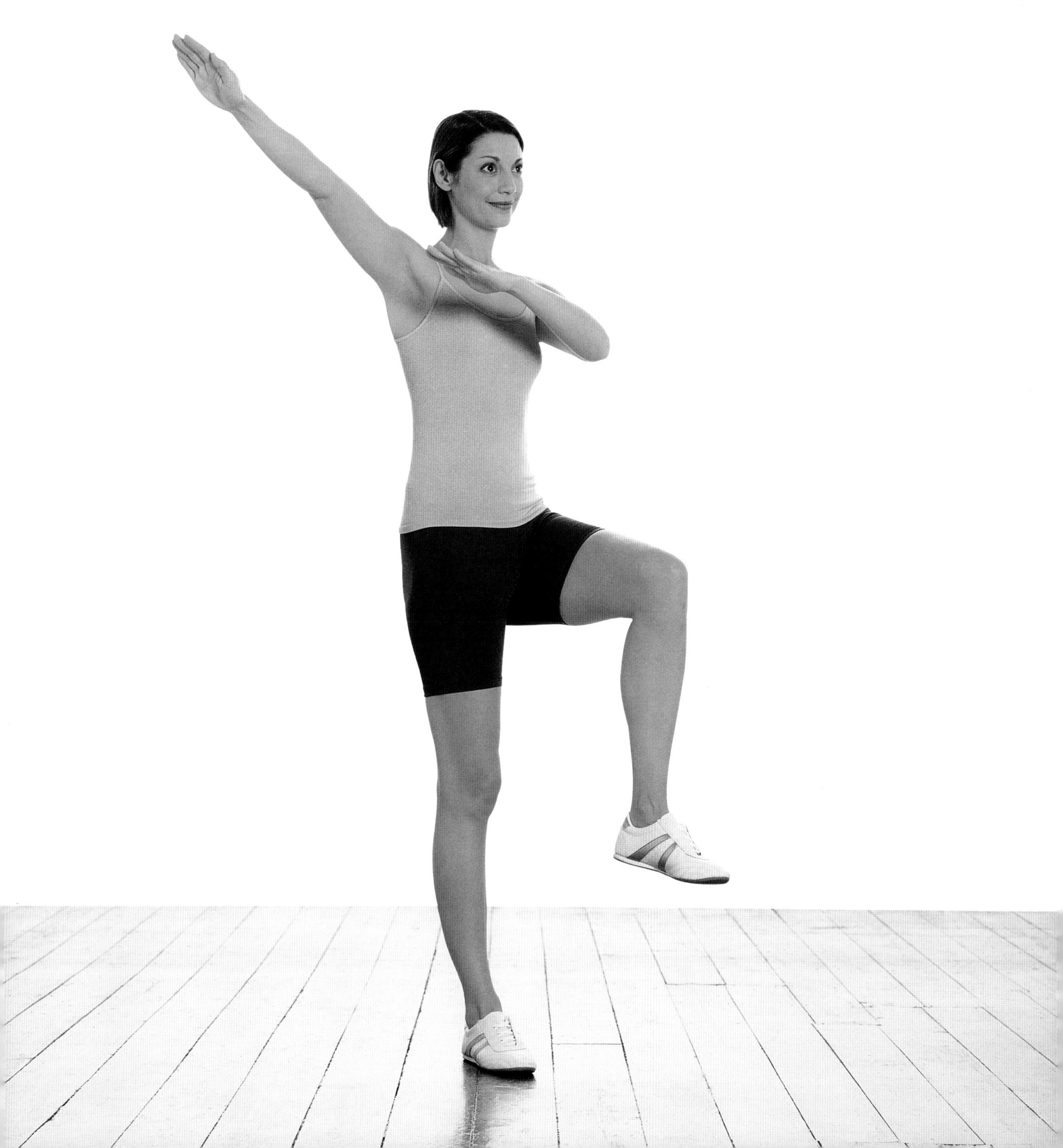

Tricep dips

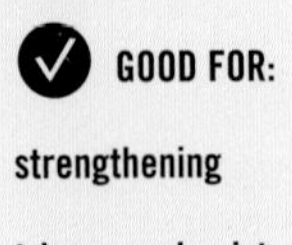

21

GOOD FOR: strengthening triceps and wrists

TAKE CARE IF: you suffer from shoulder joint or wrist problems

SEE P.90

Sit on the edge of a chair and place your hands on the seat with your fingers over the edge and your elbows pointing backward. Lift your bottom off the seat and walk your feet 1 step forward. Position your knees above your ankles with your feet parallel and hip-distance apart. Lower your bottom toward the floor by bending your elbows. Straighten your arms to bring your hips back to the starting position. Take 2 counts to lower your body and 2 counts to lift. Do 16 to 20 repetitions, or if that's too many for you, just do as many as you can.

NOTES

This exercise works the muscles at the back of the upper arm and the rear of the shoulder. The other muscles around the shoulder joint and the shoulder girdle assist in stabilizing the shoulder joint and the back while the movement takes place. As the triceps get stronger through lifting and lowering the weight of the body, the shoulder and back muscles get stronger at holding the shoulder girdle in the desired position. Focus on keeping your chest open and your shoulder blades pressing down so that your shoulders don't round forward. Your elbows should continue to point backward as you do the movement. When your arms are straight, ensure the elbows are slightly bent so that you are not locking and overloading your joints.

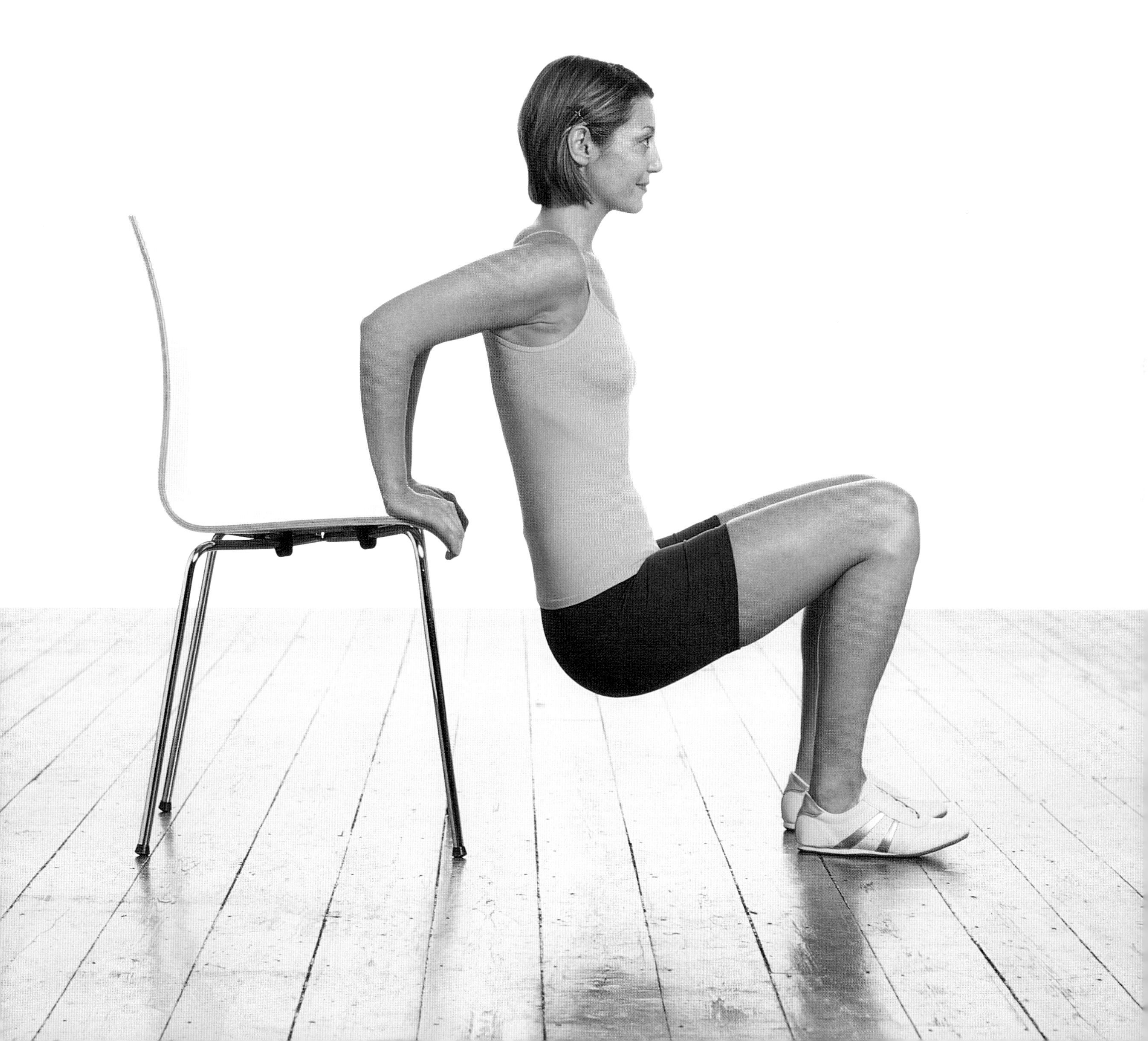

Prone leg lift

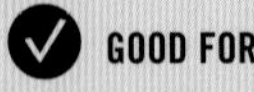

GOOD FOR:

better posture;

stronger gluteals

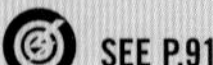

SEE P.91

Lie face down on the floor and allow your forehead to rest on the backs of your hands. Contract your deep abdominal and pelvic floor muscles and ensure your pelvis is in a neutral position. Position your legs and feet hip-distance apart. Keep your hip bones in contact with the floor and your knee straight as you contract your right buttock muscle to lift your right leg off the floor. Replace your right leg and lift the left one. Take 2 counts to lift the leg and 2 counts to lower. You can also hold the lift for 4 counts to emphasize the contraction phase. Repeat 12 to 16 times on each side.

NOTES

This exercise strengthens the gluteal muscles of the bottom. These are the largest muscles in the body and help with walking and stepping movements, as well as assisting us in standing up.

Check that your hips stay in contact with the floor throughout the exercise. To ensure this happens, consciously press them into the floor.

Although the focus is on the legs, don't forget to keep your shoulder blades drawn down your back.

You can either alternate your repetitions or you can do all the repetitions on one side and then do the other side. The latter is probably the more difficult option as the muscles don't get as much rest.

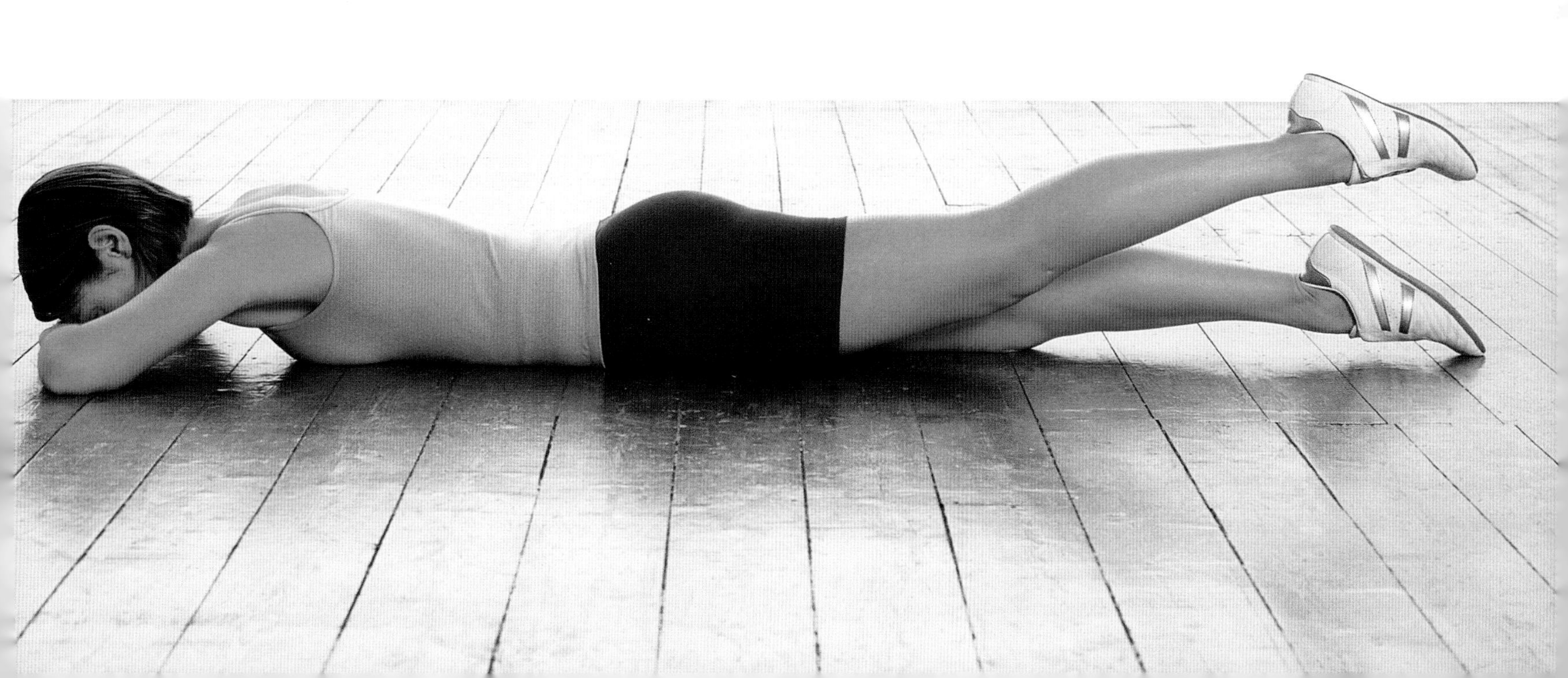

Press-ups

GOOD FOR:
core stabilization; natural synergy and coordination of the muscles, joints and nervous system of the upper body

TAKE CARE IF:
you have any shoulder or elbow issues

AVOID IF:
you suffer from acute wrist problems or osteoporosis of upper body

SEE PP.92–3

Start in an extended position on your hands and toes. Your arms should be slightly wider than your shoulders. Your fingers face forward with your shoulders, elbows and wrists in line. Keep your elbows very slightly bent. Contract your core muscles. Bend your elbows and lower your body toward the floor. When your elbows are in line with your shoulders, push yourself back up by straightening your arms. Keep your head aligned with your spine. Take 2 counts to lower your body and 2 counts to push back up. Try to do 8 to 12 repetitions as a starting point and work up to 16 repetitions.

NOTES

The press-up is a great compound exercise for the chest, arms, back and torso as all these muscles are either moving, assisting the movement or holding part of the body in position. Check that you maintain a straight line from your ear lobe, through your shoulder, hip and knee joints, to your ankle bone. The whole body should lower and lift in one piece. This exercise is good for ensuring you can work with your own body weight before concentrating on external resistance, eg using dumb-bells or weighted bars. And it can highlight the weak areas that may need some additional, specific strengthening or stretching work.

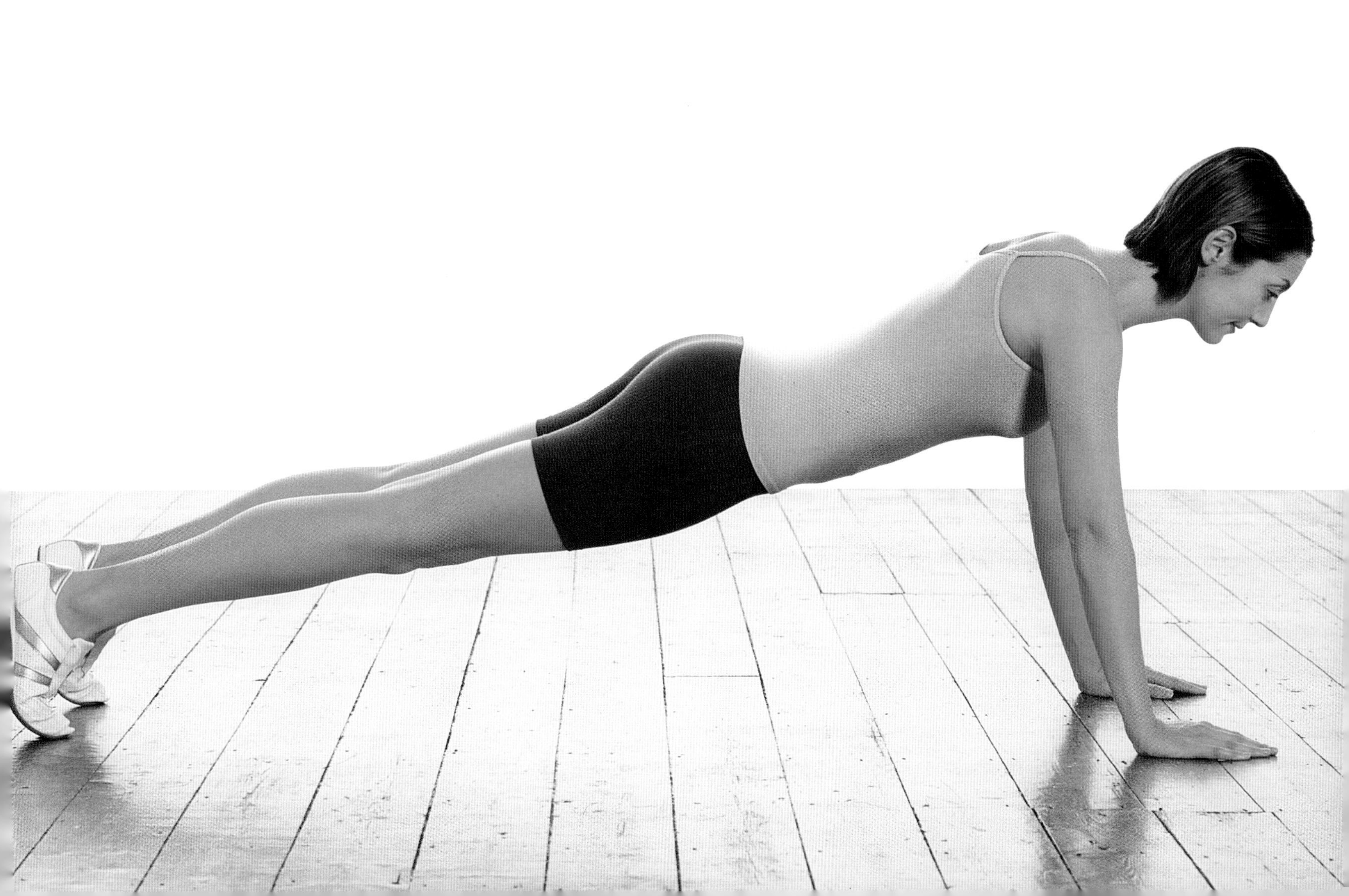

Back extension (arms by side)

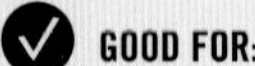

GOOD FOR: upper and lower back strength; improved synergy and coordination of back muscles

TAKE CARE IF: you suffer from disc problems

SEE PP.94–5

Lie on your stomach with your forehead resting on a folded towel. Place your arms by your side with your palms facing the ceiling. Your legs should be hip-distance apart and your feet parallel. Roll the shoulders back and down, pulling your shoulder blades toward your waist. Lift your chest off the floor, keeping your head in exactly the same position in relation to your neck and shoulders as it was when you were lying flat. Rotate your shoulders so that the palms of your hands face the sides of your thighs. Release and return to lying flat. Take 4 counts to lift and 4 counts to release. Repeat 12 to 16 times.

NOTES

This movement should activate the mid and lower fibres of the upper back. Poor posture and hours spent sitting at desks have meant that it is common for the upper back and the neck to be overworked (hence tightness and tension in these areas) and the mid back to be inactive. Pressing your shoulder blades downward should engage the mid and lower muscle fibres and have them contribute more to the work.

As you roll your shoulders back you will be encouraging the chest to open. When you hold this position as you lift the chest, you will be training the chest, shoulders and upper back to be in a good postural position.

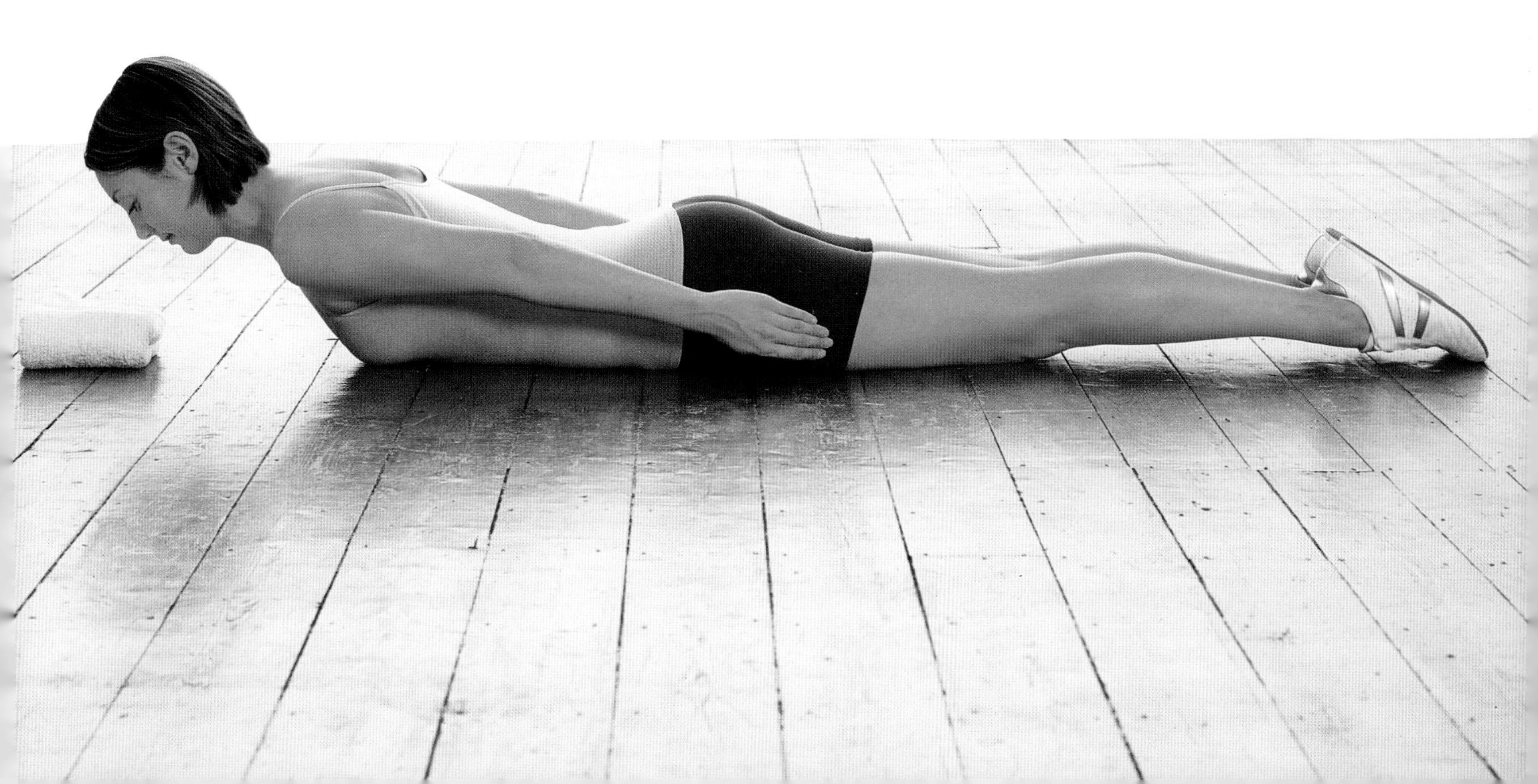

Hamstring curls (on all fours)

25

GOOD FOR: strengthening the hamstrings and buttock muscles; shoulder joint integrity; and core stabilization

TAKE CARE IF: you suffer from acute wrist problems. You can rest on your forearms and still do the exercise

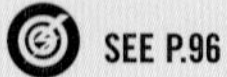

SEE P.96

Kneel down and place your hands on the floor level with your knees. Your wrists and elbows should be directly under your shoulders and your knees directly under your hip joints. Engage your core muscles. Your spine and pelvis should be in a neutral position. Lift your right leg straight out behind you, so that your knee is horizontal with your hip. Hold your thigh still and bend your knee, taking your heel toward your bottom. Then straighten your leg out. Do 16 to 20 repetitions with each leg, taking 4 counts to bend and 4 counts to straighten.

NOTES

The hamstring muscle located at the back of the thigh causes this movement to happen. At the same time, the gluteus maximus (the largest buttock muscle) works to hold the hip joint open and the leg up. As you bend the knee and bring the heel toward your bottom, you may feel a lengthening in the front of the thigh (quadriceps). The gluteus medius helps keep the pelvis level and still. And the core muscles should be switched on. This will also help strengthen the torso.

Watch that your head stays aligned with your spine and that your chin does not drop toward your chest. Keep a long spine, including your neck. Check that you have a very slight bend in your elbows. You may have to work quite hard at keeping your pelvis from twisting or dropping to one side, especially as you become more tired.

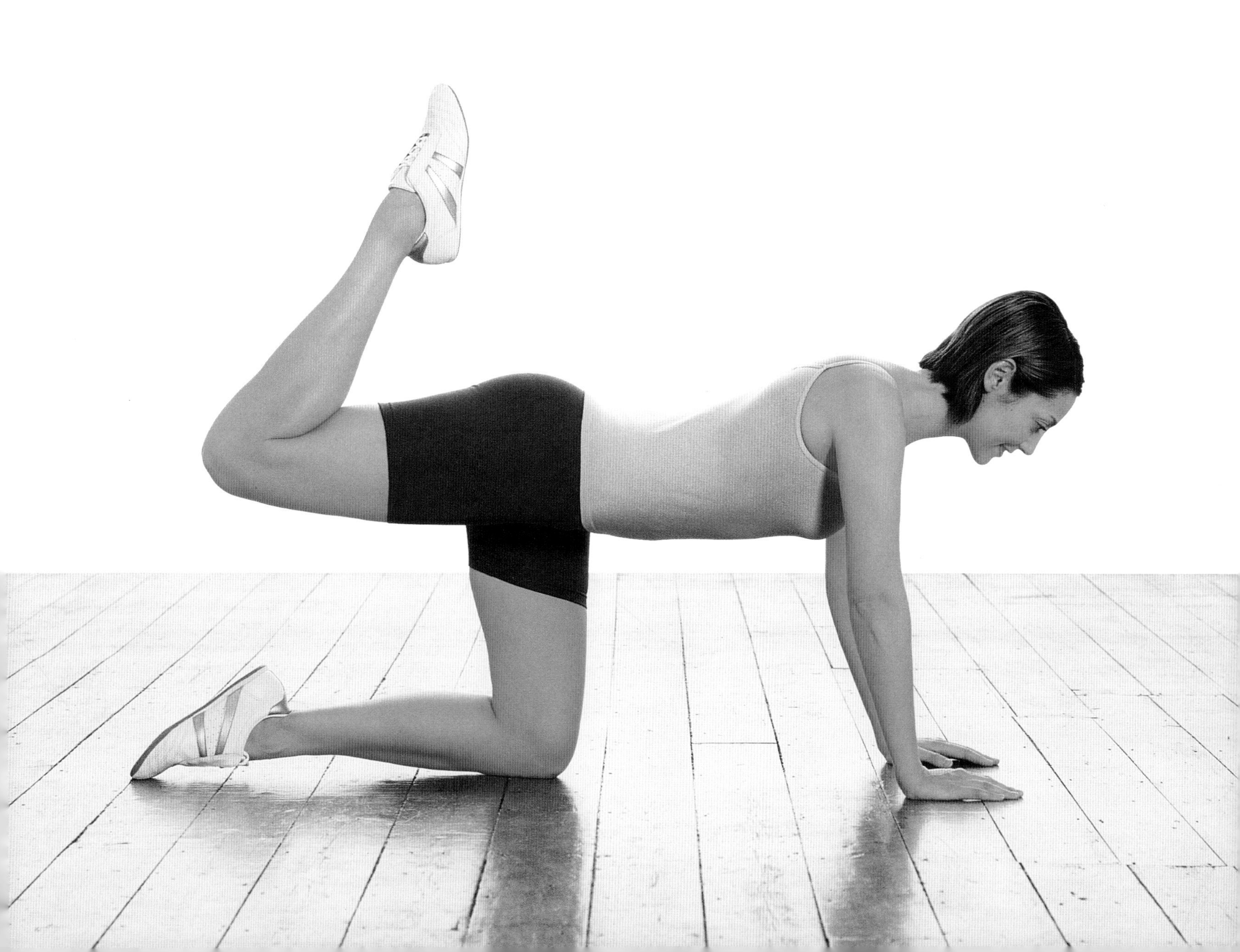

Modified "T" stand

GOOD FOR: working on core stabilization in a side lying position and for taxing and improving the integrity of the shoulder joint

TAKE CARE IF: you have any shoulder joint issues

SEE P.97

Lie on your right side and prop yourself up with your forearm resting on a folded towel. Ensure that your elbow is directly under your shoulder. Have your legs straight out with the foot of your top leg just in front of the foot of your bottom leg. Align your pelvis so that your left hip is above your right and have your knees and ankles as level as possible. Take 2 counts to lift your hips off the floor, so that your body is in a straight line from ear to ankles. Lower your hips back to the floor in 2 counts. Repeat 8 to 12 times, then change to the left side.

NOTES

This movement works on strengthening the shoulder joint by putting the muscles, bones and nerves under pressure of some body weight. It also works a muscle around the waist (quadratus lumborum) that assists with stabilization of the pelvis and torso. This muscle helps keep you upright and balanced when you are carrying a heavy bag in one hand. Ensure that your core muscles, pelvic floor and transversus abdominus muscles are engaged (see p.19). This will also help with stabilization.

Try to keep your head central – don't let it drop to the lower shoulder. Roll the shoulders back and press the shoulder blades down to prevent the top shoulder from rounding forward. Concentrate on lengthening through both sides of your torso.

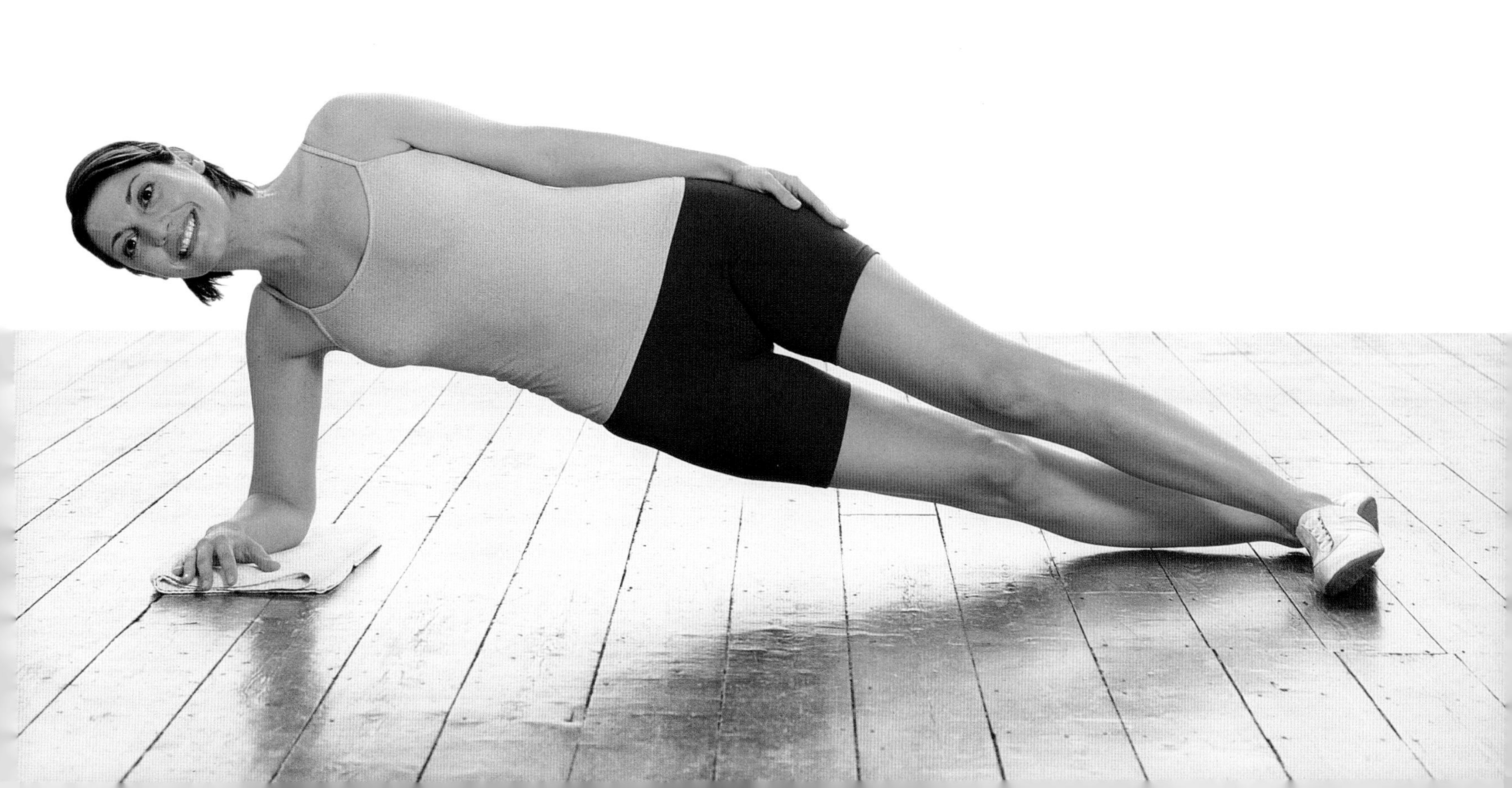

Bridge

GOOD FOR: combining mobility with stability (strength) as they should complement each other; mobilizing the spine; core stability

SEE PP.98–9

Lie on your back with your knees bent. Have your knees and feet hip-distance apart. Place your arms by your side, palms upward. Start with your spine in neutral (there should be a small gap between the floor and the natural curve of your lower back). Slowly tilt your pelvis backward and press your lower back into the floor. Roll through your spine, lifting each vertebra off the floor in turn. Stop when your body weight is across your upper back and shoulders, and hips and knees are in line. Hold for 3 breaths. Lower your body back to the floor, vertebra by vertebra, rounding through your spine. Repeat 5 times.

NOTES

This is a combined mobilization and strengthening exercise. The mobilizing movement (the rounding up and down) helps address stiffness in the back.

The strengthening part of the exercise (the hold at the top) involves the whole body. Check that your knees stay in place, your heels are close to your bottom and your feet are still parallel. Use your inner and outer thigh muscles to hold your legs still. Your pelvis should also be held still and positioned so that your hip bones are level and not tilting to the right or the left. Focus on keeping your hips open, and don't let your bottom drop. Check that your shoulders are away from your ears.

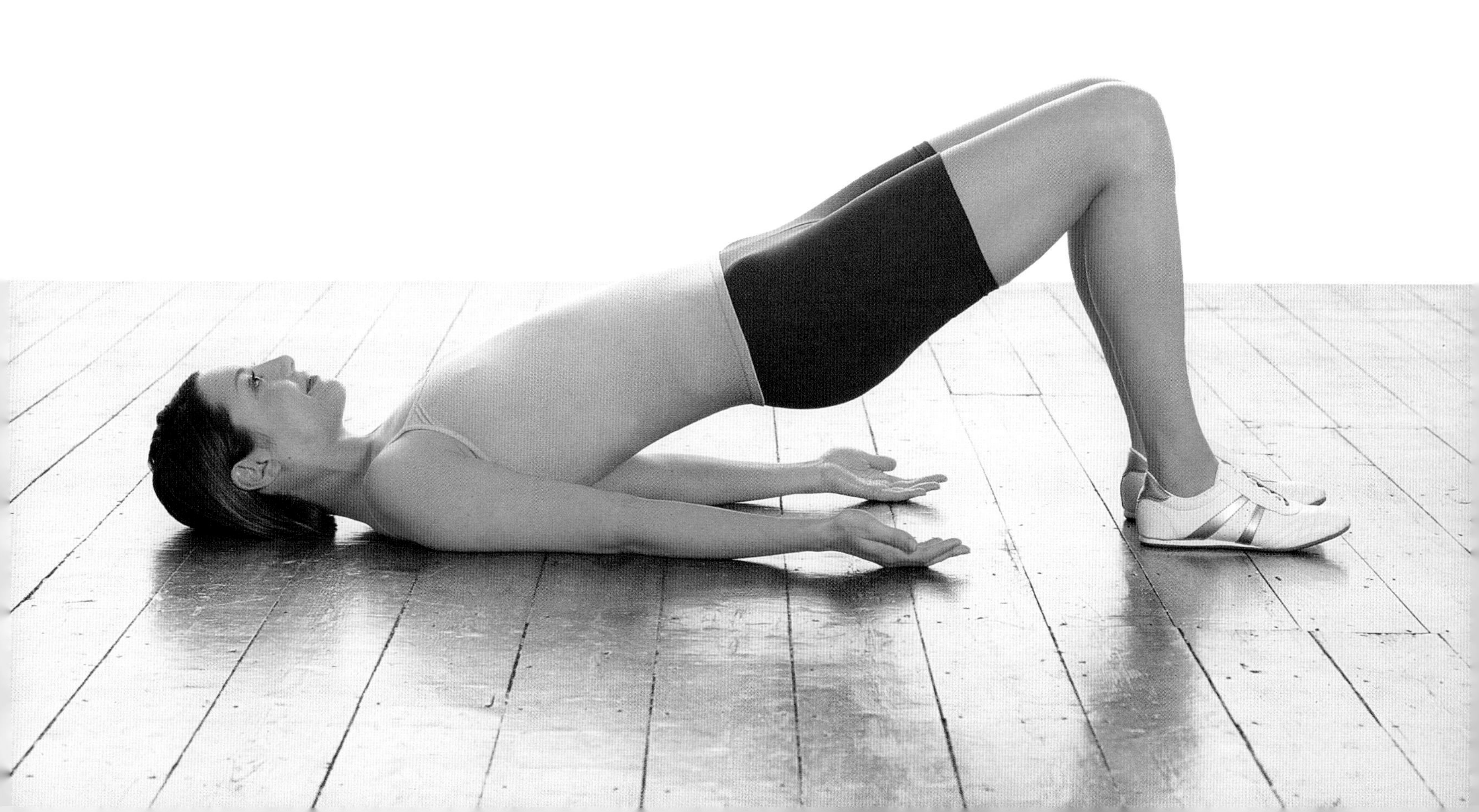

Lying hamstring with calf and hip flexor stretch

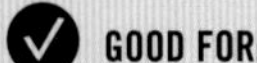

GOOD FOR:

a time efficient stretch that targets a selection of different muscles; runners and sports people

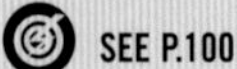

SEE P.100

Lie on your back with your legs hip-distance apart. Relax your upper body and draw your shoulders away from your ears. Raise your right leg so that your foot is toward the ceiling. Use your hands to hold your leg in place. Straighten out your knee joint as much as possible. Press your heel toward the ceiling and pull your toes toward your nose. Your left leg should be straight with the back of your knee pressing toward the floor. Hold for 4 to 6 deep, relaxing breaths. Then change sides.

NOTES

This is a combination stretch for the hamstring and calf muscles of the raised leg and the hip flexors (the muscles that run across the front of your hip) of the other leg. This stretch is great for creating synergy between muscles that work together or affect the working of one another.

The aim of this stretch is to lengthen the muscles and also to relax them. For example, hamstrings are often tight and shortened in people who sit for long periods. Try not to bend your knee to bring your thigh closer to your chest, as this will turn off the hamstring stretch. If straightening your knee means your leg moves further away from your chest and it becomes difficult to hold, place a towel around your leg and hold onto the towel instead of your leg.

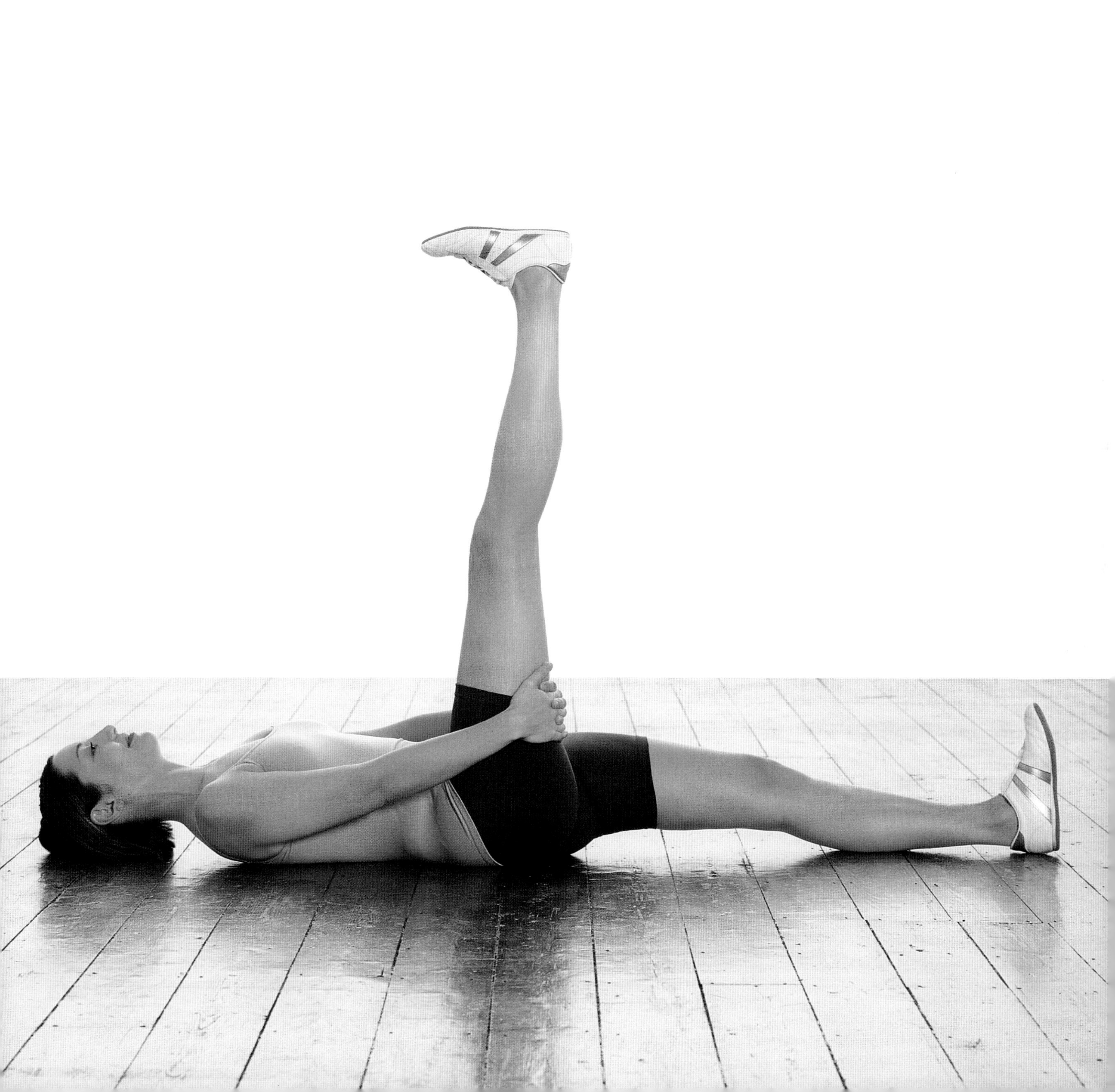

Gluts and chest stretch

GOOD FOR: addressing rounded shoulder posture or lower body postural issues caused by a stiff lower back or tight gluteals

SEE P.101

Lie on your back with your legs stretched out along the floor. Stretch your right arm out to the right side so that it is in line with your right shoulder. Bend your right knee into your chest and use your left hand to gently pull your knee over to the left side until you feel a stretch in your right hip/buttock. Look toward your right hand. The back of your right shoulder must stay in contact with the floor and you should feel a stretch across the right side of your chest and right shoulder. Hold this position for 4 to 5 deep breaths. Gently release and change sides.

NOTES

The aim of this stretch is to open up the chest and shoulder joint. This will help with mobility of the shoulder joint and better upper body posture. When the leg is taken across the body, ensure that the back of your shoulder remains in contact with the floor and that your whole chest points up to the ceiling, rather than twisting to either side. If your shoulder starts to lift it will be easier to get your knee across, which will reduce the effectiveness of the stretch.

When people stand with their feet turned out it can often be because their gluteals and external rotator muscles (that cause the leg/hip joint to turn out) are tight. This stretch can lengthen these muscles and allow a more neutral, parallel position to be adopted through the hips and feet.

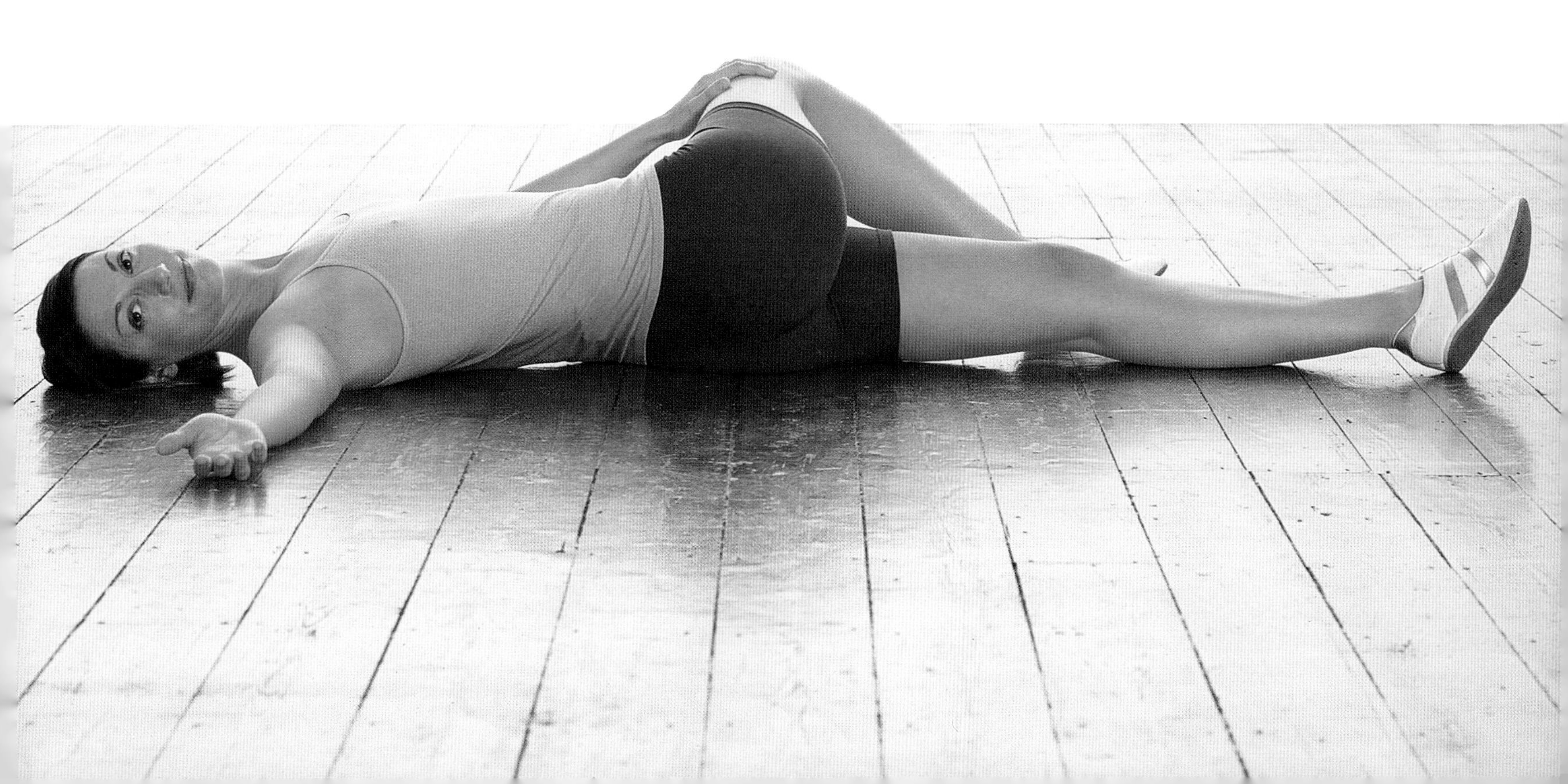

Side-lying quad with hip flexor stretch

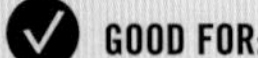

GOOD FOR: addressing tightness in the front of the thighs and hips and associated postural issues

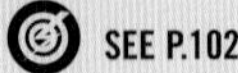

SEE P.102

Lie on your right side with your head resting on your right arm and your legs stretched out along the floor. Bend your left knee and draw your heel up toward your bottom. Your left knee should be above and in line with your right knee. Hold the lower shin, ankle or foot of your left leg. Tilt your pelvis backward by pushing your hips forward. You should feel a stretch through the front of your left hip and down the front of your left thigh. Hold the position for 4 to 5 deep breaths. Release and repeat the stretch on your right side.

NOTES

The hip flexors cause the body to bend at the hip, and so straightening out or opening the hips will stretch and lengthen this muscle group. The quadriceps cause the knee joint to extend or straighten out, and so the reverse action of bending the knee will stretch these muscles.

Keep your lifting knee in line with your hips and parallel with your other knee. If you feel a good stretch when holding onto your shin/ankle/foot, don't progress to tilting your hips and easing your knee back. Just enjoy the stretch in this first position.

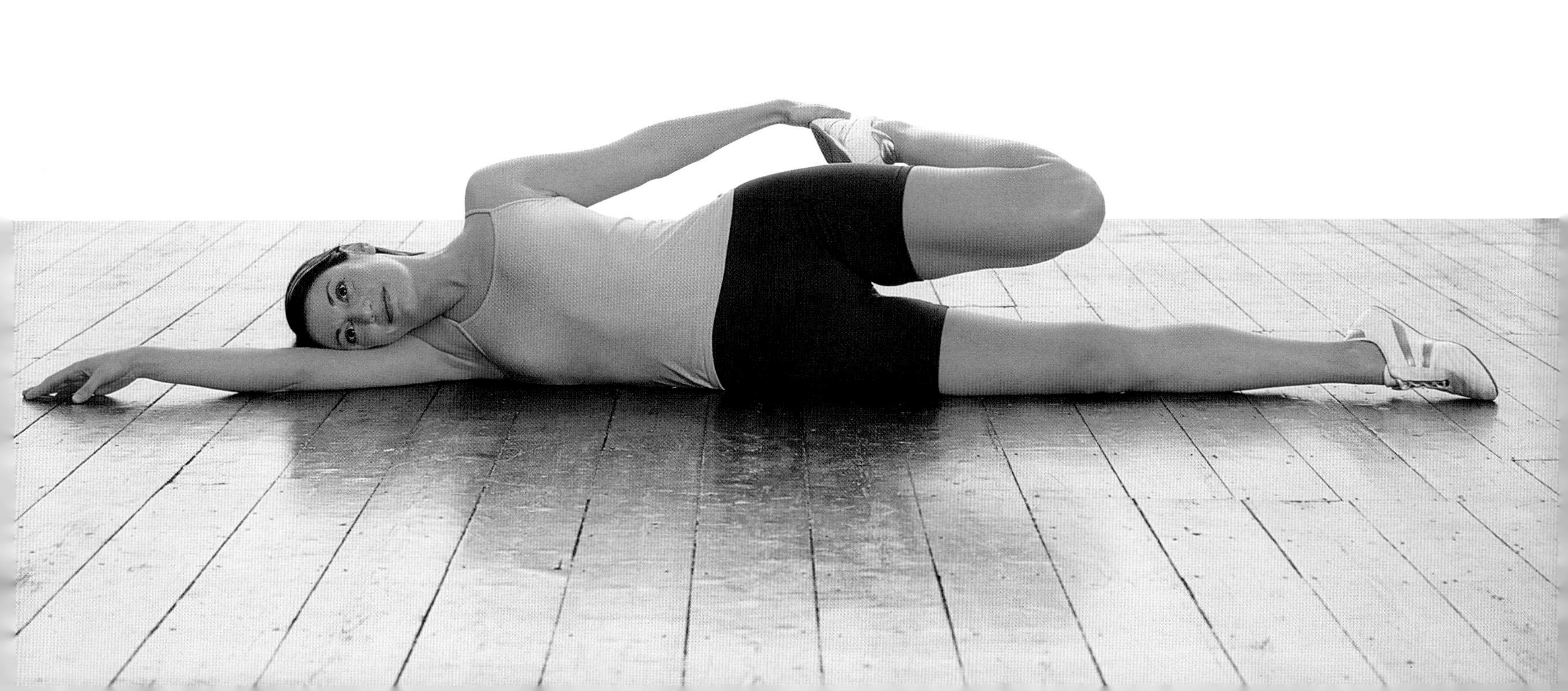

Lateral stretch

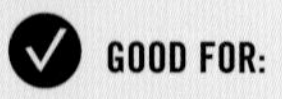 GOOD FOR:
lengthening the torso

TAKE CARE IF:
you have knee problems (ensure that you use a towel under your supporting knee) or wrist problems

SEE P.103

Kneel on a mat or a towel and place your left hand out to the left side in line with your left knee. Your fingers should be pointing out to the side. Extend your right leg out to the right side keeping your foot facing forward. Press the sole of your right foot into the floor. Lift your right arm overhead so that your fingers point to the left. Your palm should be facing the floor. Press your left hip forward to lengthen your quadriceps. Hold the position for 4 to 5 deep breaths. Release and repeat the same stretch on your left side.

NOTES

This is another great combination stretch that hits a number of different muscle groups at once. How you feel this stretch will depend on which of your muscles are tight, shortened, or have good flexibility.

Pressing the foot of the extended leg into the floor can give a mild stretch along the outside of the ankle joint. The main stretch is along the torso – it should feel as if you are lengthening out of your hips. The "lats" should feel a stretch because the arm is extended overhead and you may also feel a stretch along the inner thigh of the extended leg. Try to lengthen through your elbow, wrist and fingers to experience a feeling of total stretch. Check that your shoulders are not touching your ears. You should still think about drawing your shoulders down.

Watch that you have not dropped your head toward your lower shoulder.

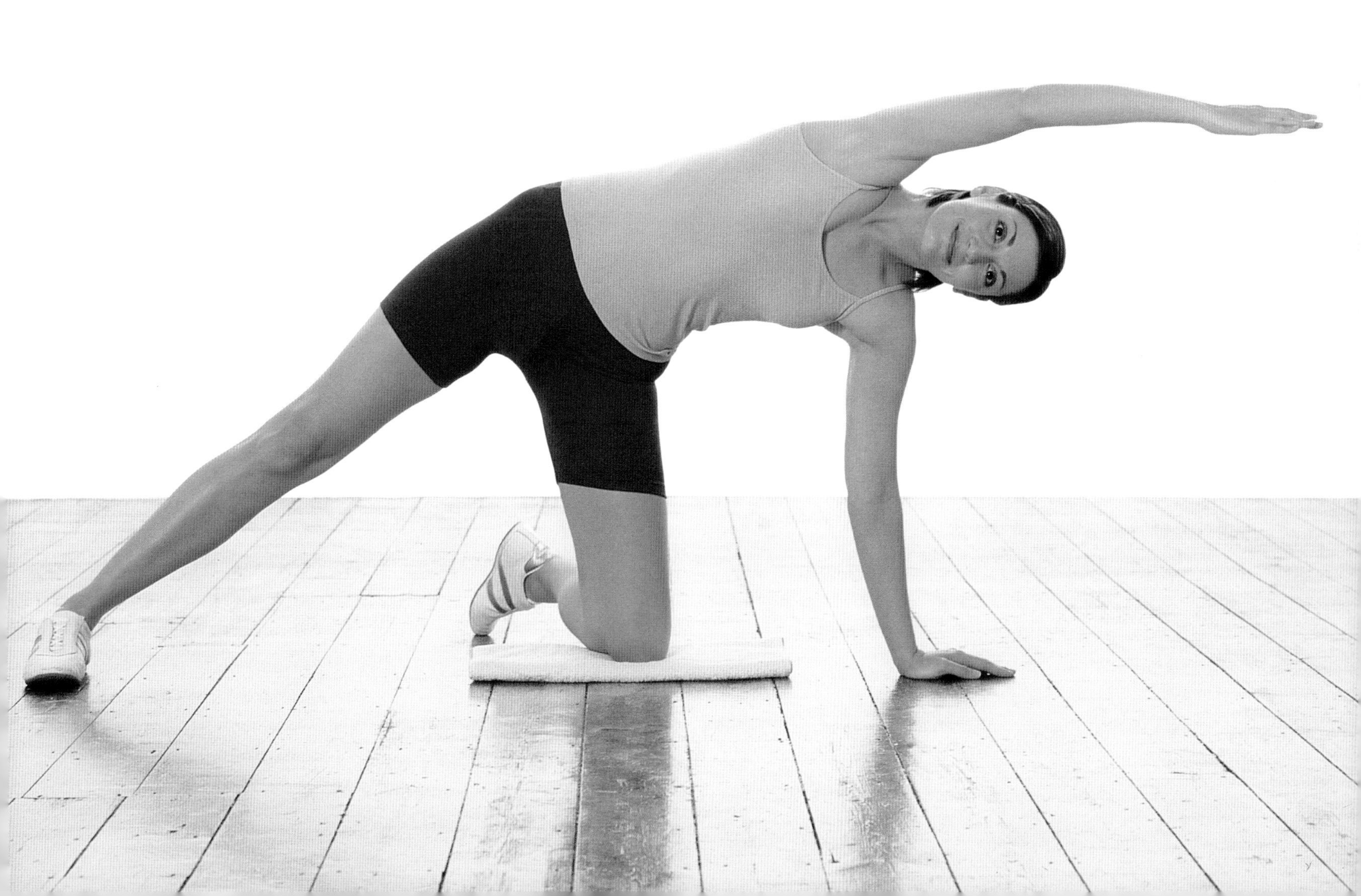

Cat stretch

32

GOOD FOR: lengthening the back after exercise; ending a workout if there is no time for relaxation

TAKE CARE IF: you have wrist problems (support yourself on your fists) or disc problems

SEE P.104

On a mat or a folded towel, kneel on all fours with your knees in line with your hips and your wrists and elbows in line with your shoulders. Your fingers should be facing forward. Check that your spine (and head) is long and in a neutral position before you start. Tilt your chin toward your chest and gently round your back from the base of your skull to your tailbone. Hold the position for 4 to 6 deep breaths. Release and repeat the same stretch another 3 times.

NOTES

This is a great stretch for the whole back and the neck. It can also be used to work on mobility of the spine. Think of your spine as a chain: you should be able to bend that chain at each link (although there is less movement in the lower back and where the vertebrae are fused).

You can do the Cat Stretch starting from your neck and head, rounding through each vertebra until you get to your tailbone or you can start at your tailbone and work your way up to your neck and head. Isolating the movements in this fashion can make you aware of tight spots along your spine that could benefit from specific, focused mobility exercises.

Try to keep your legs in the same position throughout the stretch and avoid rocking your pelvis from side to side. If resting on your wrists is uncomfortable, make your hands into fists and rest on these instead.

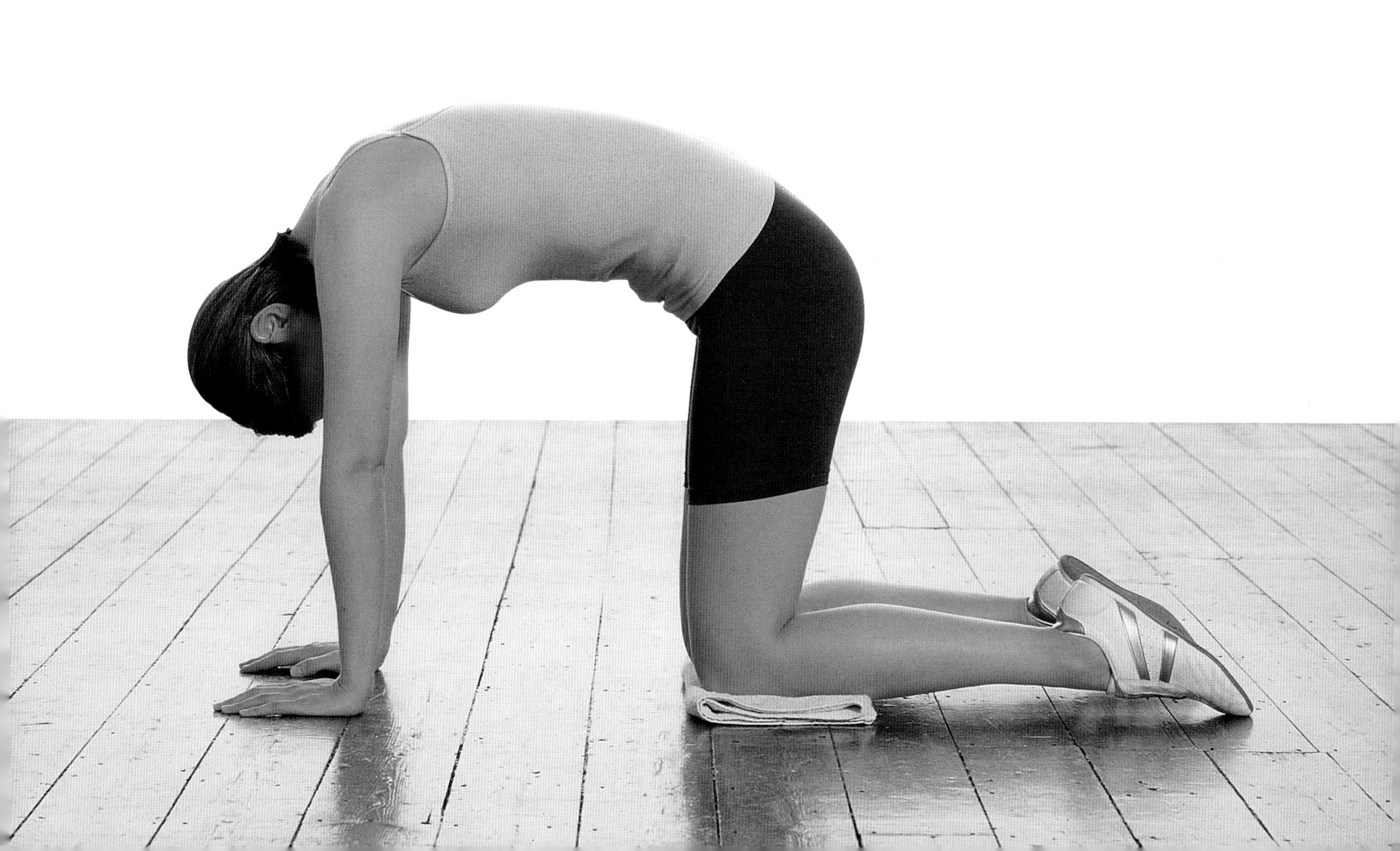

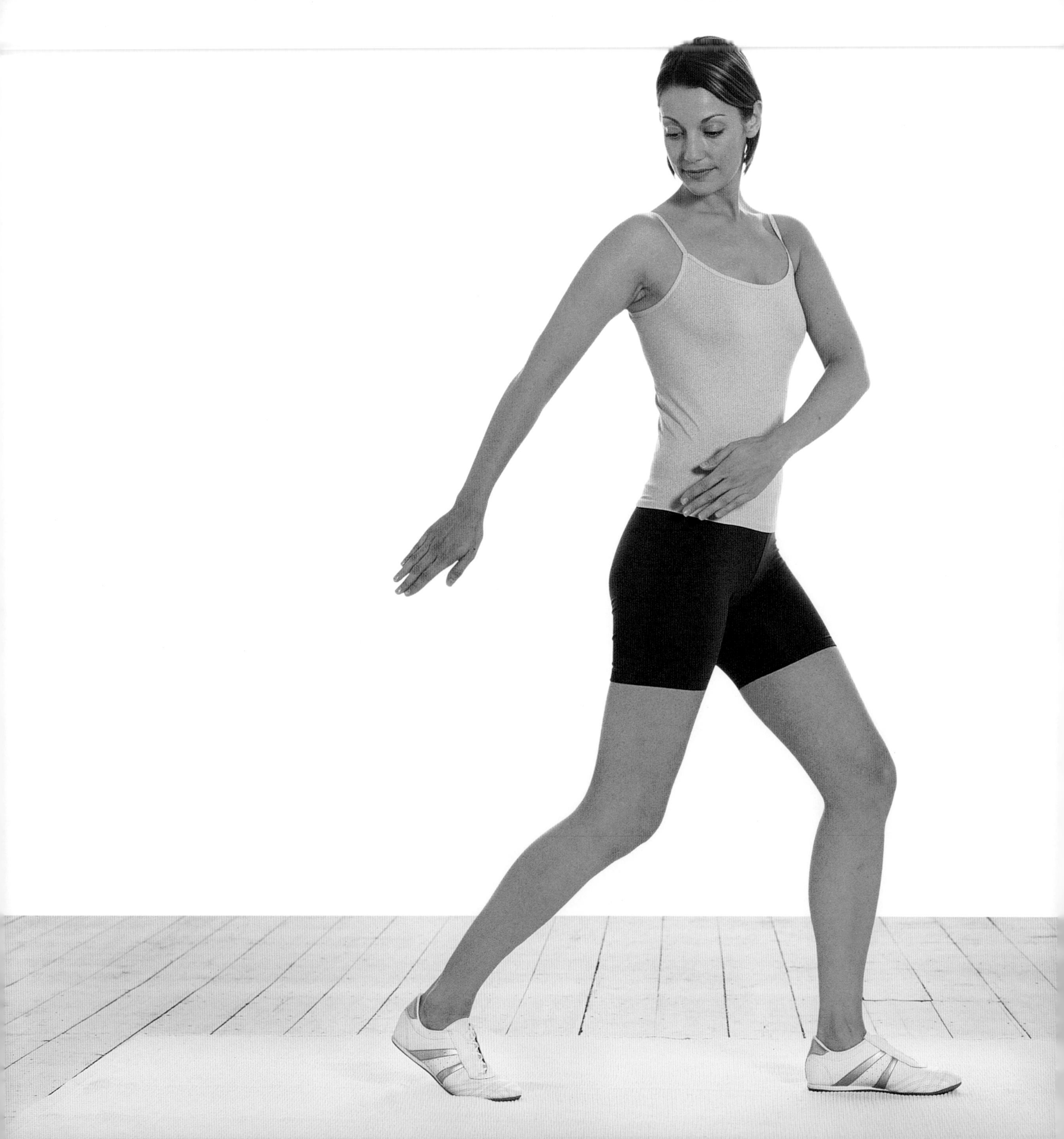

CHAPTER 3: Easy Solutions

When devising any fitness training programme I take a number of things into account. An individual's age, and more importantly, health, fitness and skill levels all need to be considered and acknowledged because they may affect which exercises can be done or how a particular exercise should be done. This Easy Solutions chapter does just that. Exercises can always be modified to meet your specific physical requirements and so if there are any exercises in Chapter 2 that cause you concern you can turn to this section to find a solution to suit you.

Some of the exercises have more than one solution. These double as exercise progressions, and you can work through them one at a time until you are ready to tackle the target exercise. However, if a muscle, bone or nerve issue means that the target exercise is inappropriate for you, stick to the solution exercise. This means that you will still be safely working the relevant muscle, bone or nerve.

Easy fitness, safe fitness

It is important to monitor your workout to ensure you are not working too hard, but that you are working at a level that will make the workout effective and cause the desired improvements in the body.

The different fitness components are measured differently. Cardiovascular exercise is often measured by heart rate and wearing a heart rate monitor is the most accurate way to do this. If you do not own a heart rate monitor, a common and easy method of monitoring that you can use is called “Rate of Perceived Exertion”. You answer the question “how hard do you think you are working on a scale of 1 to 10?”– 1 being that the exercise takes very little effort and 10 being that you have to stop this second because you are too tired to carry on. In order to gain health benefits, you should be working between 3 and 6 (moderate to hard). For fitness benefits, you should aim to work the whole range between 3 and 9/10 (moderate to very, very hard). This is a subjective method that takes account of how you feel on any particular day. If you are tired, stressed, lacking energy, etc this will affect the way you feel and how you gauge your level.

Strength is measured by how much weight you can lift or, as is the case in this book, whether you can complete the repetitions with good form and technique. Your aim is to reach a point where your muscles are tired and struggle to do the last few repetitions.

Flexibility is measured by the angles of joints and the position of certain body parts as you do a stretch, and by how you feel the stretch. If you don't feel a stretch you are probably not in quite the right position unless you are very flexible. For example, always double check that your shoulder stays in contact with the floor in the Gluts and Chest Stretch (pp.68–9). Different people will feel the stretches in different places depending on how tight certain muscles are. The intensity of a stretch may differ depending on whether you are stretching your right side or your left side.

Always monitor what you are doing and how you are doing it. Work to your own pace and build up slowly. Remember that this Easy Solutions Chapter is here to help you do that. Be aware of how you feel and never work through pain. If pain persists you should visit a medical practitioner about the problem.

If you have not exercised for a while or if some of the exercises are new to you, you might experience Delayed Onset Muscle Soreness (DOMS). This is the discomfort you feel the day after exercise, or even the day after that. Don't panic! Usually, this is simply the muscles reacting to new or unaccustomed activity and the discomfort will normally subside within a few days. However, some signs that you might be overdoing things are constant tiredness, lack of energy and persistent or frequent injuries.

Step-ups with chest press

SOLUTION

Using your arms and legs in specific patterns can challenge coordination and cause frustration when your limbs don't seem to want to work smoothly together. Don't give up! Keep trying to master the pattern as coordination is a skill that can be trained like any other skill.

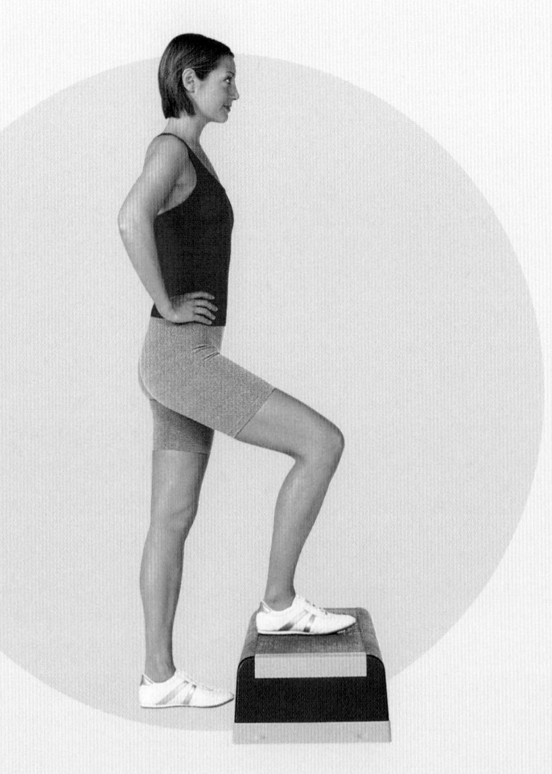

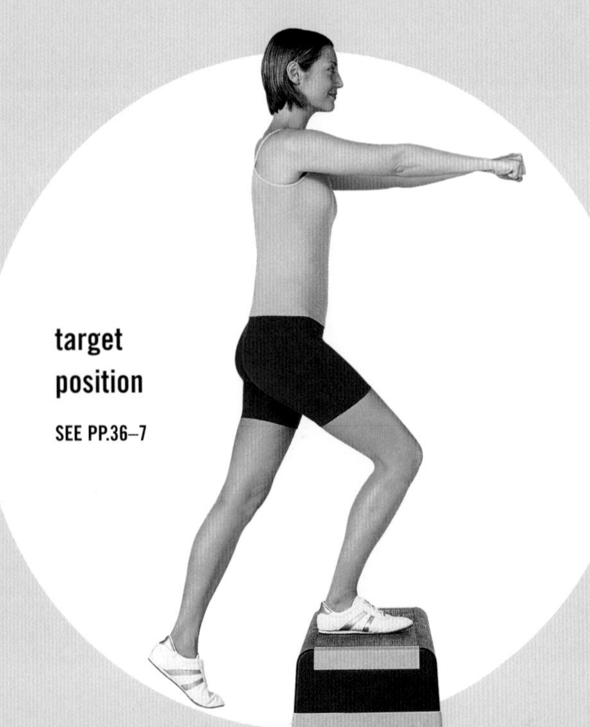

target position

SEE PP.36–7

PROBLEM: **I can't coordinate my arms and legs.**

SOLUTION: **Do the Step-ups with your hands on your hips. You can also try doing the arms while stepping up and down on a lower step and at a slower pace, but bear in mind that this will affect the intensity of the exercise.**

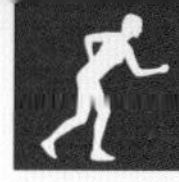

Sprint-runs

SOLUTION

Sprinting may seem quite taxing and hard work if you have not exercised for a while. The easiest way to modify this exercise is to reduce the pace so that you are jogging, power walking or even walking on the spot.

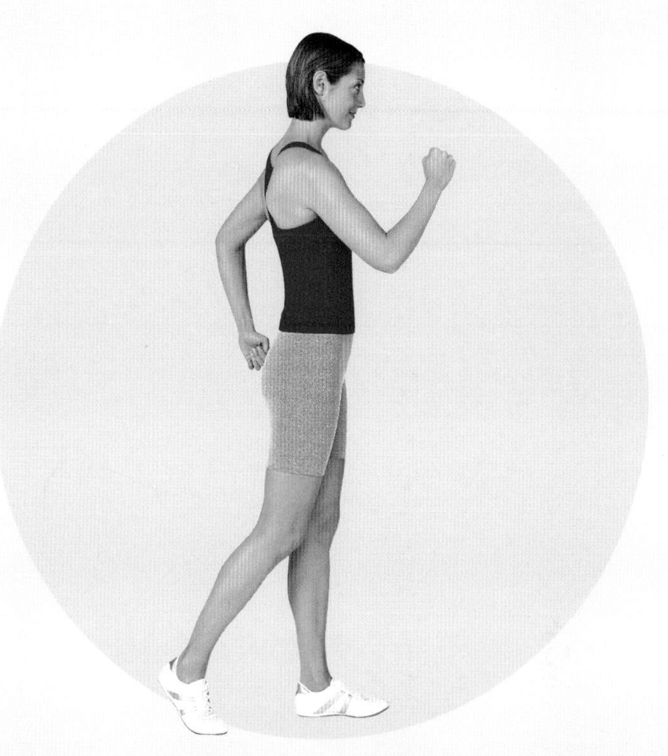

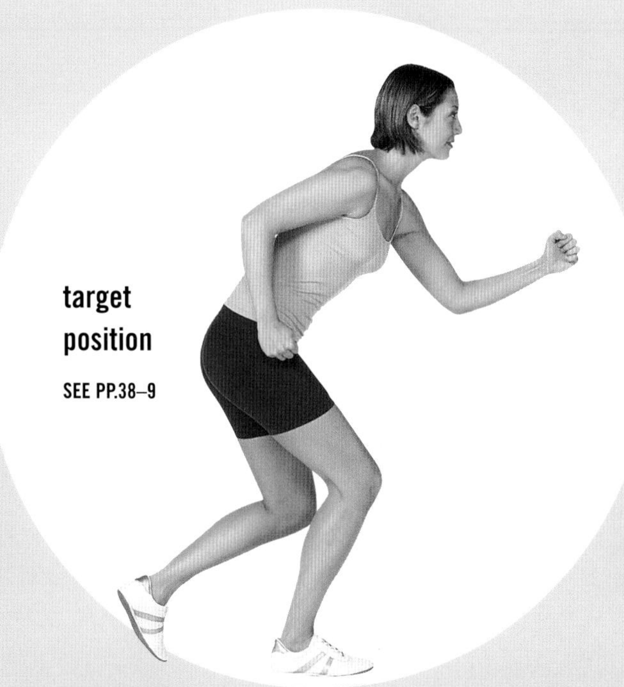

target position

SEE PP.38–9

PROBLEM: **The sprints are too much for me. I find them very hard to do.**

SOLUTION: **March on the spot, taking the intensity higher by lifting your knees and really pumping your arms as you march. You can then progress to marching from marker to marker as fast as you can.**

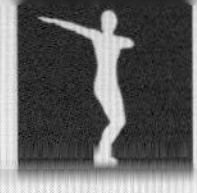

Jumping twists

SOLUTION

This exercise has a lot of continuous impact. If you have problems with your knees and/or ankles, and therefore struggle to perform this movement or to keep it going, or if you just can't get the twist and jump to work together, try the solution described below.

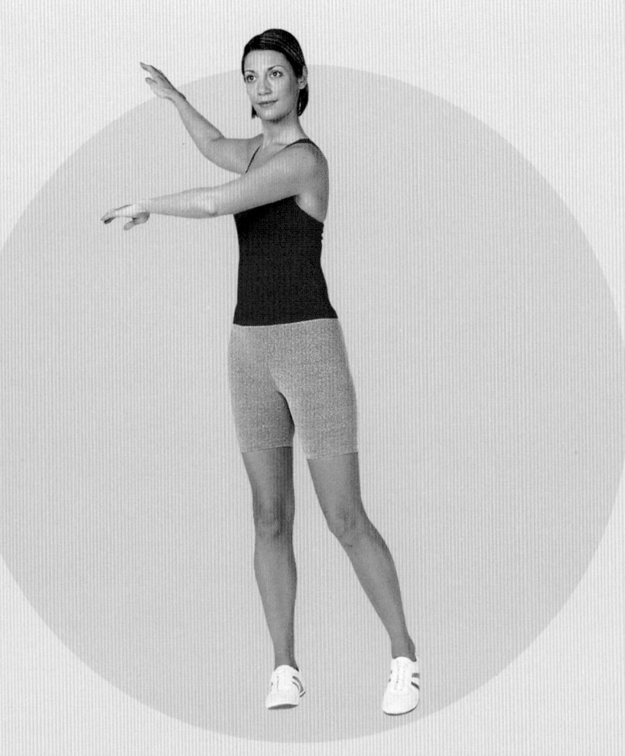

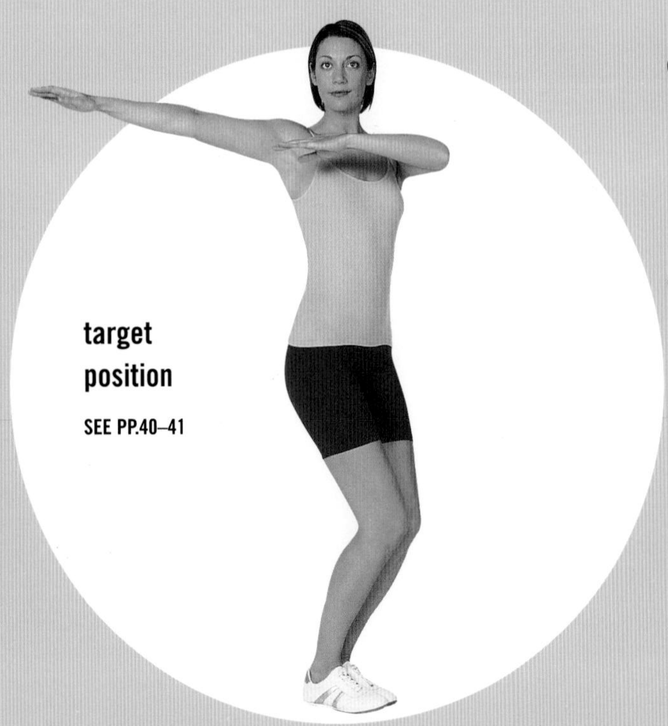

target position

SEE PP.40–41

PROBLEM: **The jumping has a lot of impact. It hurts my knees and/or ankles.**

SOLUTION: **Try doing the twisting action without the jump. Stand with with your feet shoulder-width apart. Twist your whole body from side to side, using your arms in a controlled fashion to assist the movement. As you twist to the right, allow your left heel to lift and vice versa.**

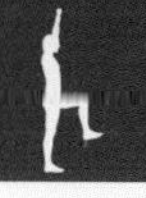

Knee lifts with arms overhead

SOLUTION

If your coordination and/or balance skills are over challenged by this movement, do only the leg action. The legs are the larger muscle group and you will still achieve reasonable intensity for cardiovascular benefits even if you don't use your arms.

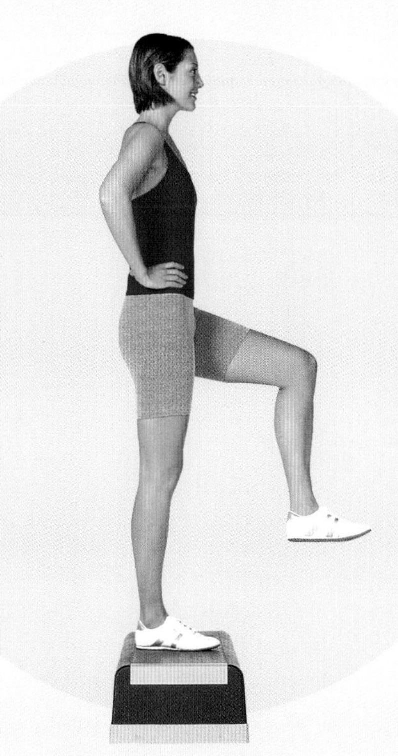

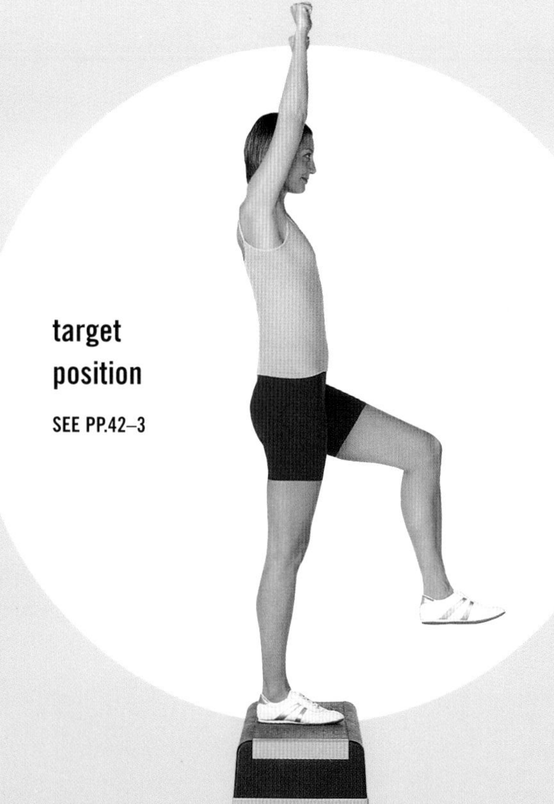

target position

SEE PP.42–3

PROBLEM: **I find using both my arms and legs too much effort and want to lower the intensity.**

SOLUTION: **Do the knee lifts with your hands resting on your hips. Focus on standing tall throughout the movement.**

Wall jumps

SOLUTION

Hip, knee and ankle issues can make the jump unsuitable for some people because of the mechanics of bending the hips, knees and ankles when taking off and the impact sustained through the joints on landing. A good, low-impact alternative is given below.

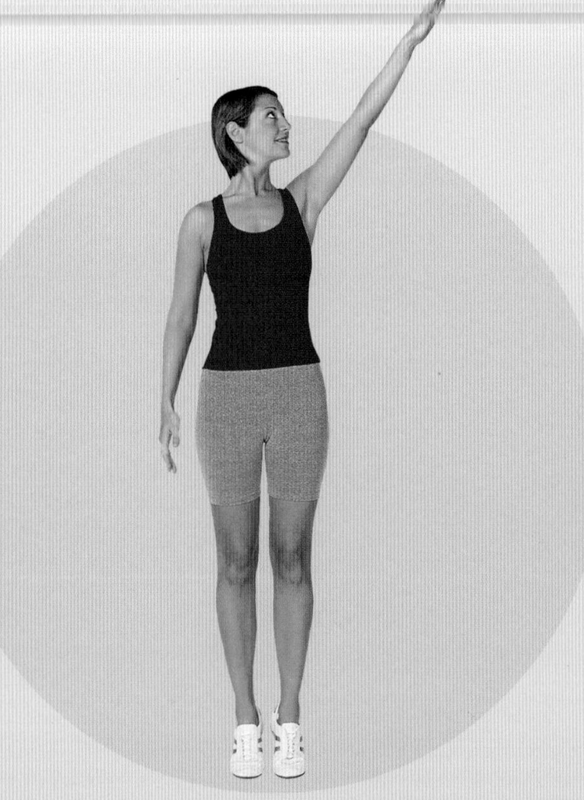

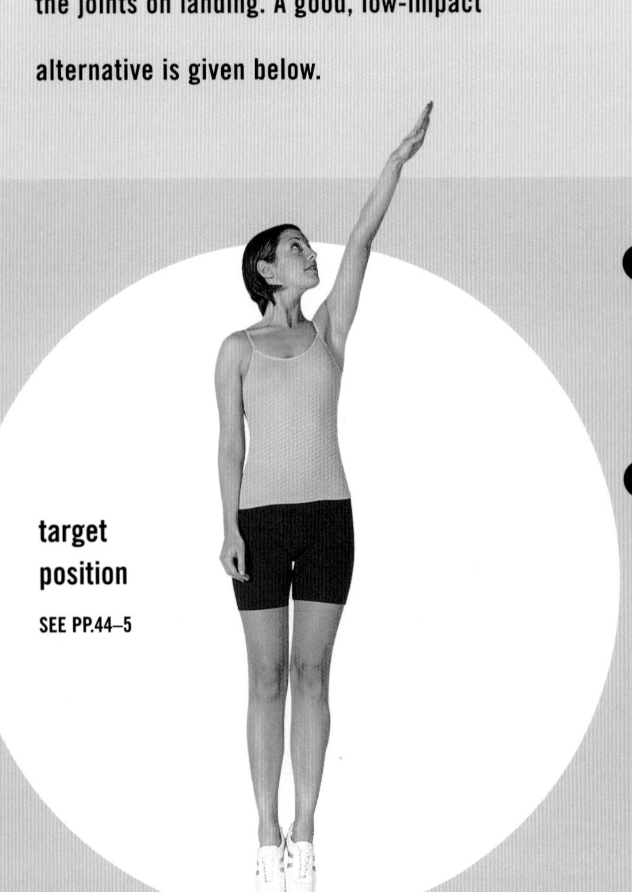

target position

SEE PP.44–5

PROBLEM: **I have trouble jumping because my joints are a bit stiff.**

SOLUTION: **Walk or run to the wall and then reach up and try to touch the imaginary spot by doing a heel raise. Lower your heels and walk or shuffle back to your start position.**

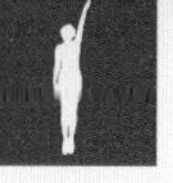

Line skiing

SOLUTION

If you need to avoid high-impact activity because of joint or bone health, or if you need to decrease the intensity of this exercise, try the following solution that is low impact and more gentle on the bones and joints.

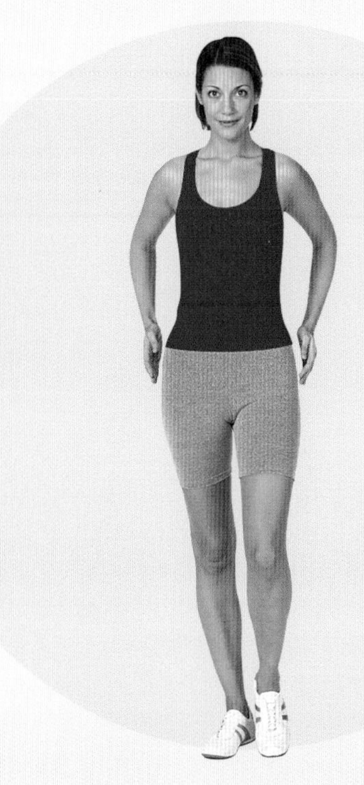

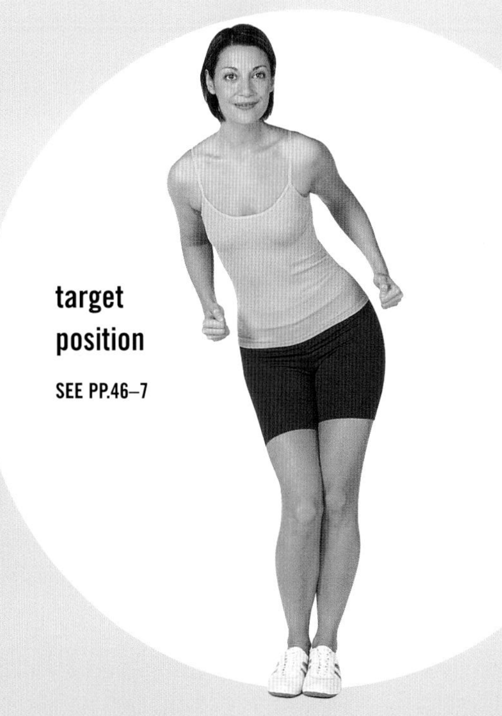

target position

SEE PP.46–7

PROBLEM: **My knees and ankles are not very stable and I would prefer not to do high-impact movements.**

SOLUTION: **Stand to the right of the line. Side step over the line with your right foot. Then step over with your left foot and tap the floor. Repeat from left to right. Use the Line Skiing arm actions as you step. Speed up the steps, but maintain good form and large arm movements.**

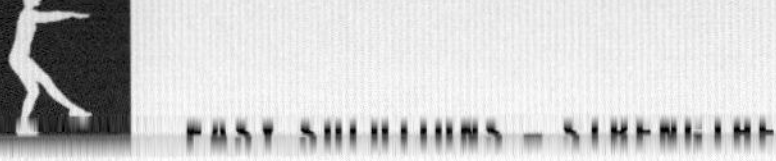

Single leg squats

SOLUTIONS

This is a demanding, integrated exercise made up of different elements that can be quite a challenge to do well. The solutions give a number of step-by-step progressions that allow you to work up to the final exercise over time.

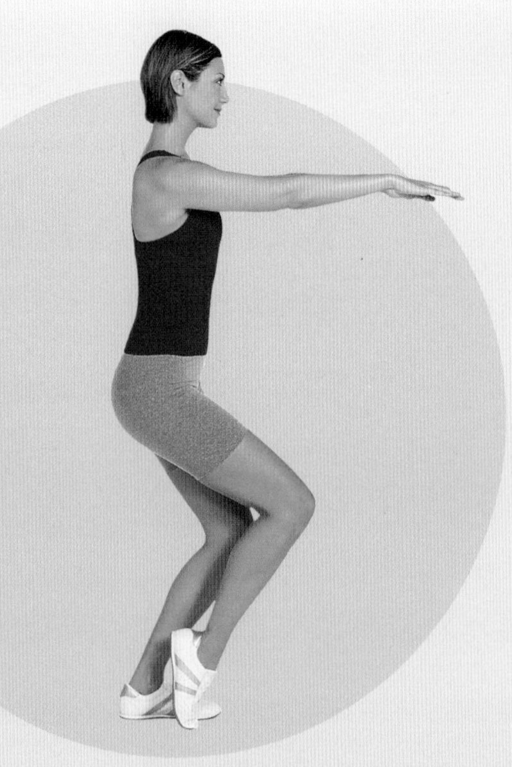

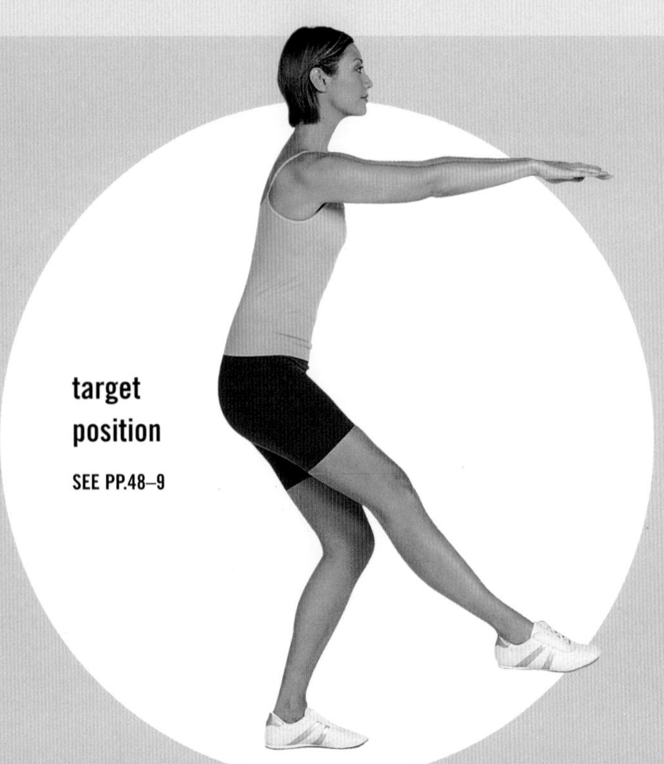

target position

SEE PP.48–9

PROBLEM: **My balance is not good and I don't feel confident standing on one leg.**

SOLUTION: **Try doing the squat without extending your leg. Instead of taking your foot fully off the floor, rest your big toe lightly on the floor to help maintain your balance as you squat.**

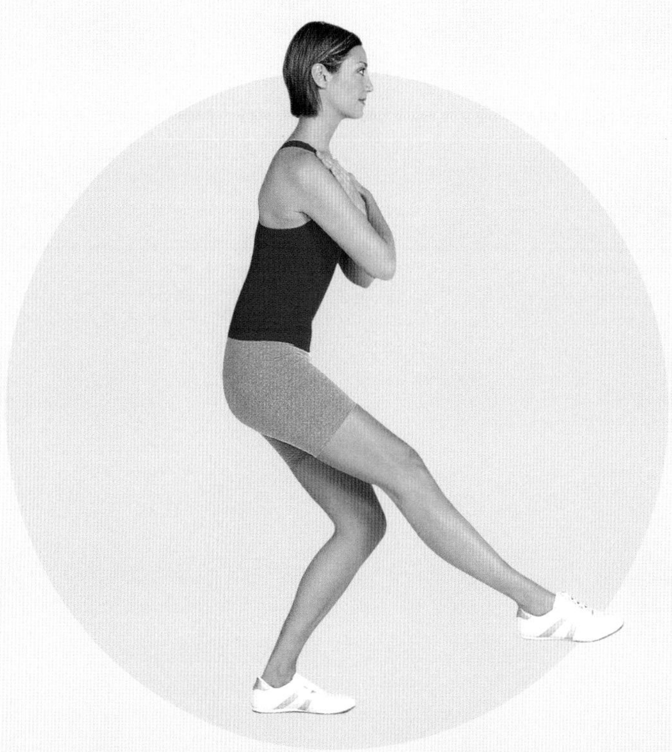

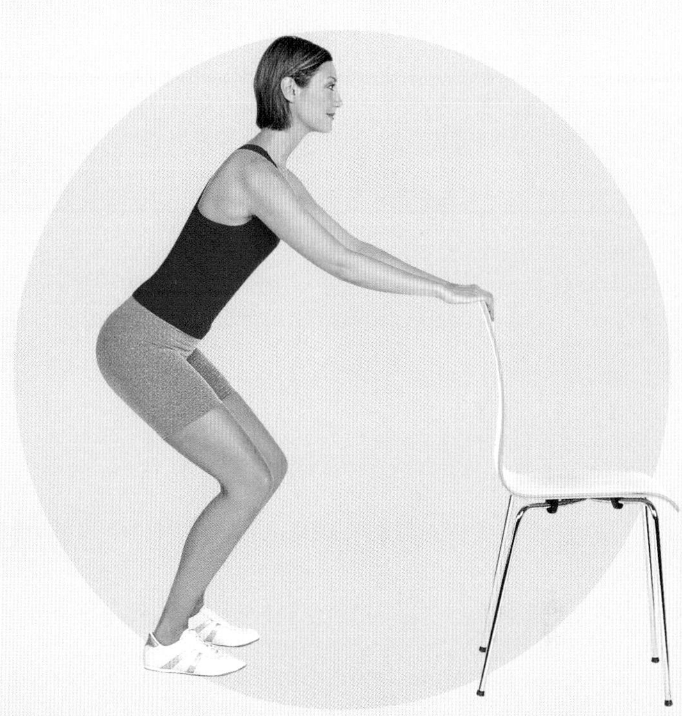

PROBLEM: **I feel shaky when I try to raise my arms and stand on one leg at the same time.**

SOLUTION: **Rest your hands on your hips, on the front of your thighs or place them across your chest. Keeping your hands and arms still and close to your body will make your squat less shaky.**

PROBLEM: **I seem to bend over too much and don't have enough strength in my upper body to maintain a strong upper body posture.**

SOLUTION: **Use a chair to support yourself as you squat. This will enable you to focus on keeping your ribs and hips the same distance apart, your back in neutral and your chest facing forward. Avoid putting too much of your weight on the chair: use it only for support.**

Lunge, knee lift and cross chop

SOLUTIONS

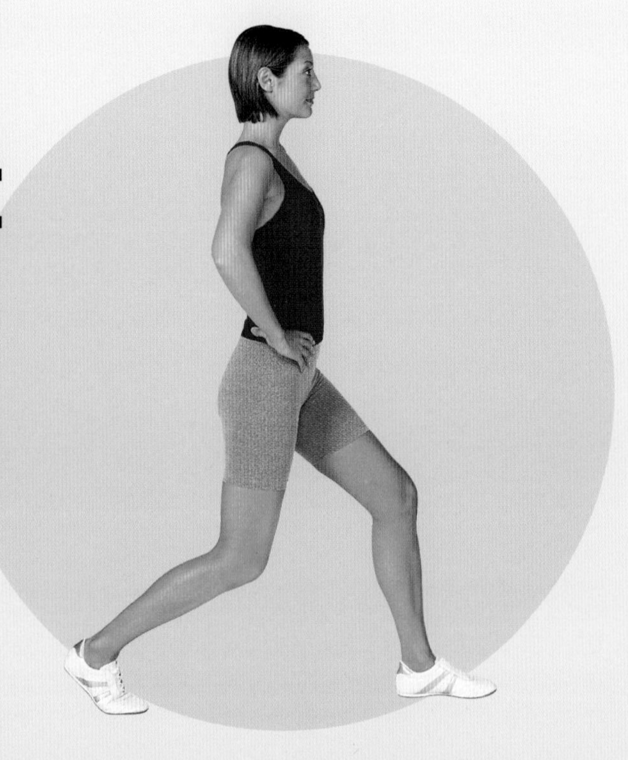

This exercise has different components that are easy to practice separately. Becoming proficient at the different parts will boost your confidence and prepare you to do the complete exercise with really good technique when you put everything together.

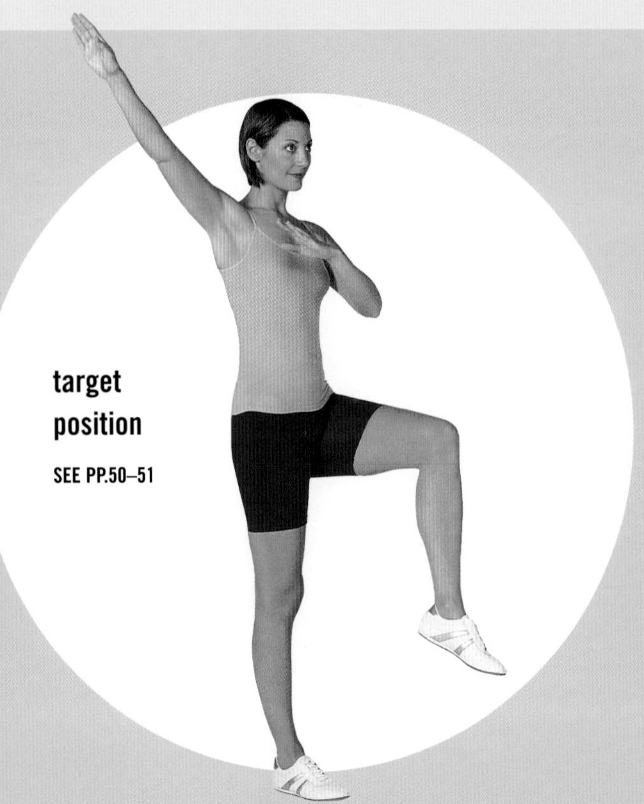

target position

SEE PP.50–51

PROBLEM: **I would like to improve my confidence doing a basic Lunge before I move on to the Knee Lift and Cross Chop.**

SOLUTION: **You can do the Lunge as an exercise on its own. Step your right foot back and with your hands on your hips, bend both knees and lower your back knee toward the floor. Press back up by straightening both legs, and change sides.**

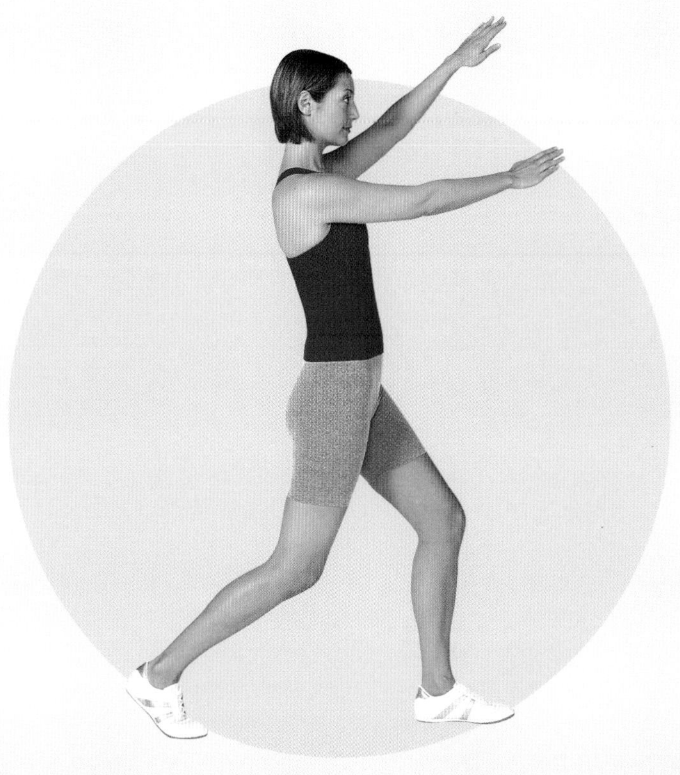

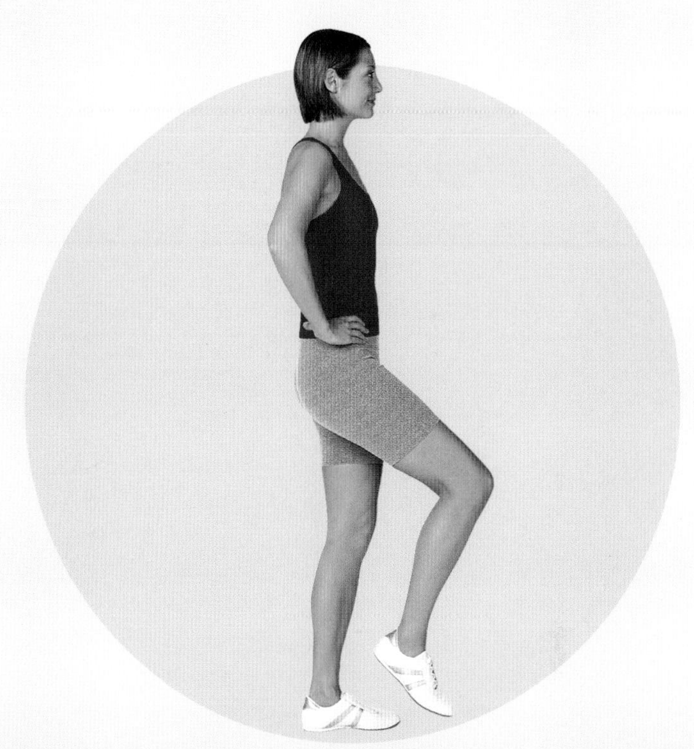

PROBLEM: **I find it awkward coordinating the arm and leg movements.**

SOLUTION: **Step into the Lunge position and just hold this stance while you do the arm movements. Pull your arms down across your body and then lift them up again along the same route. Make the arm movements as strong as you can. Initially keep looking straight ahead and then follow your fingers.**

PROBLEM: **I find it difficult to maintain my balance.**

SOLUTION: **You can only improve your balance by doing movements that require balance, so try doing the Lunge and Knee Lift without the arms. This will allow you to focus on your lower body movement.**

Tricep dips

SOLUTION

Lowering and lifting your own body weight in this exercise requires a lot of strength in the triceps and can be quite taxing on the wrists. This solution enables you to develop strength lifting and lowering your body weight at chair level where you are working against less gravity than when you are working below the level of the chair.

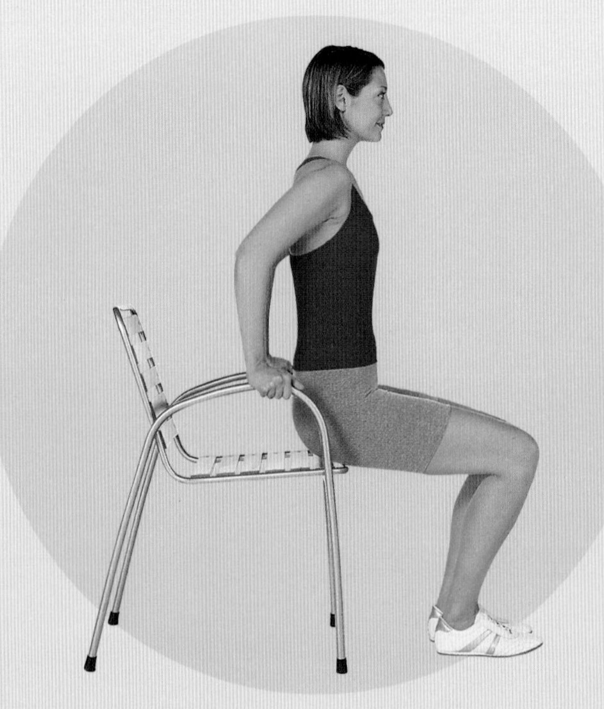

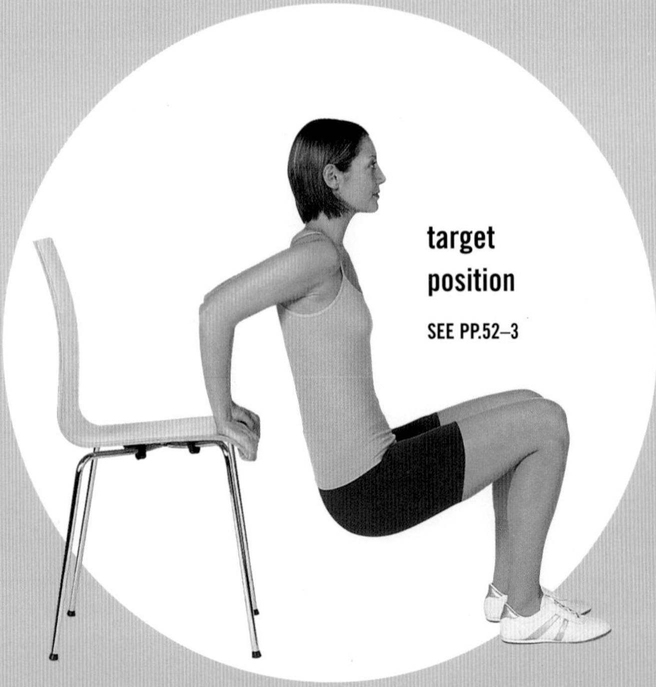

target position

SEE PP.52–3

PROBLEM: **My wrists tire quite quickly when doing this exercise.**

SOLUTION: **Sit on a chair and place your hands on the arms of the chair with your elbows pointing backward. Lift your bottom off the seat by straightening your arms without locking out your elbows. Lower yourself back down to a sitting position, reserving a little weight in your arms for the next lift.**

Prone leg lift

SOLUTION

People who sit for long periods of the day will often find that their gluteal muscles have become lazy and ineffective in their job of extending the front of the hip joint. As a result other muscles, usually the hamstrings, are overworked to compensate and this can lead to muscle imbalance.

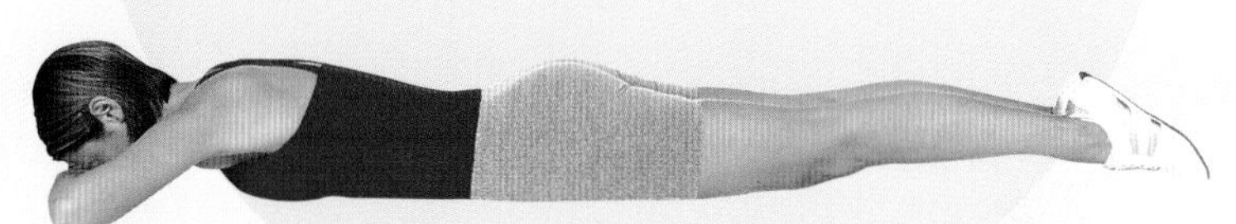

target position

SEE PP.54–5

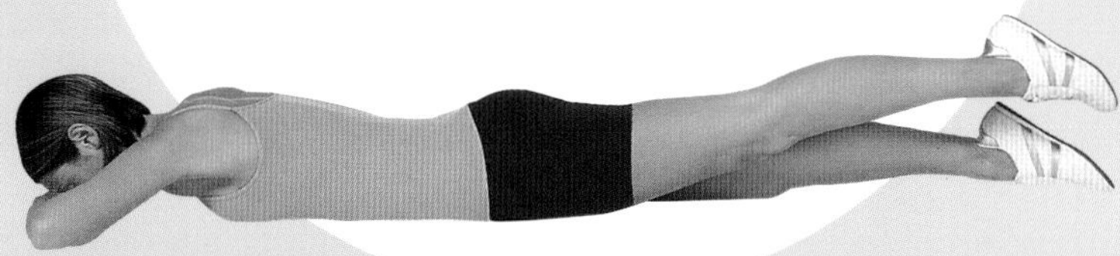

PROBLEM: **I find it hard to lift and hold my leg up while keeping my hips on the floor.**

SOLUTION: **Instead of contracting your right buttock muscle to lift your right leg, you should squeeze your buttocks together as if you are trying to hold a pound coin between your buttock cheeks. Hold the squeeze for 4 seconds and release.**

Press-ups

SOLUTIONS

Press-ups demand a lot of strength from the smaller and often weaker muscles of the arms and the back while also requiring good stabilizing strength in the torso. If you do not regularly do Press-ups or if they are a new exercise for you, it is a good idea to start with the first solution and work your way through the variations toward a good full Press-up.

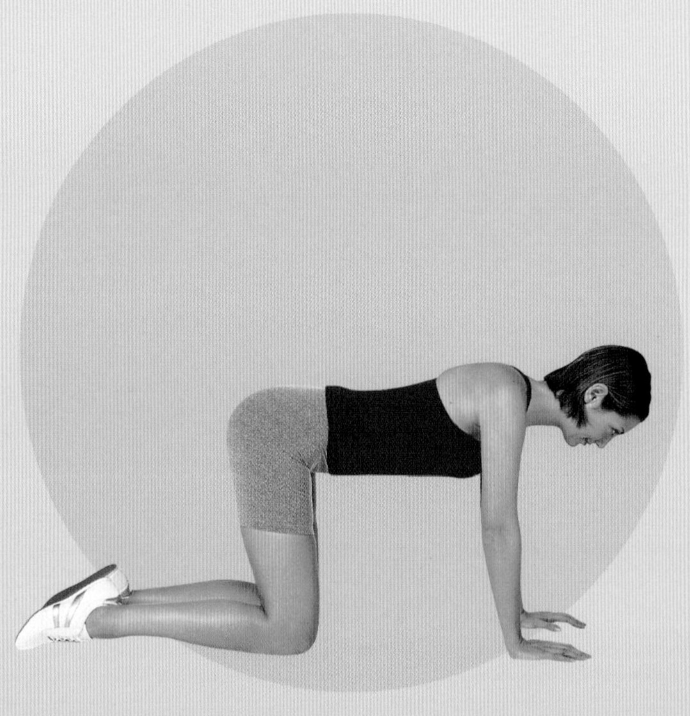

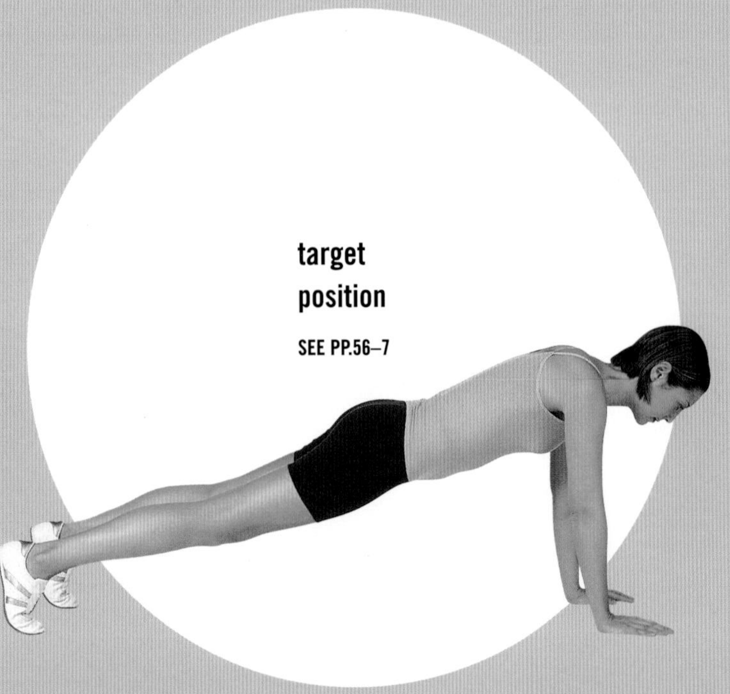

target position

SEE PP.56–7

ⓧ PROBLEM: **I have not got the strength in my arms to lower my body to the floor.**

✓ SOLUTION: **Kneel on all fours so that your knees are under your hips and your wrists and elbows are directly under your shoulders. Engage your core muscles. Hold the position for 3 deep breaths. Sit back and release your arms and then repeat.**

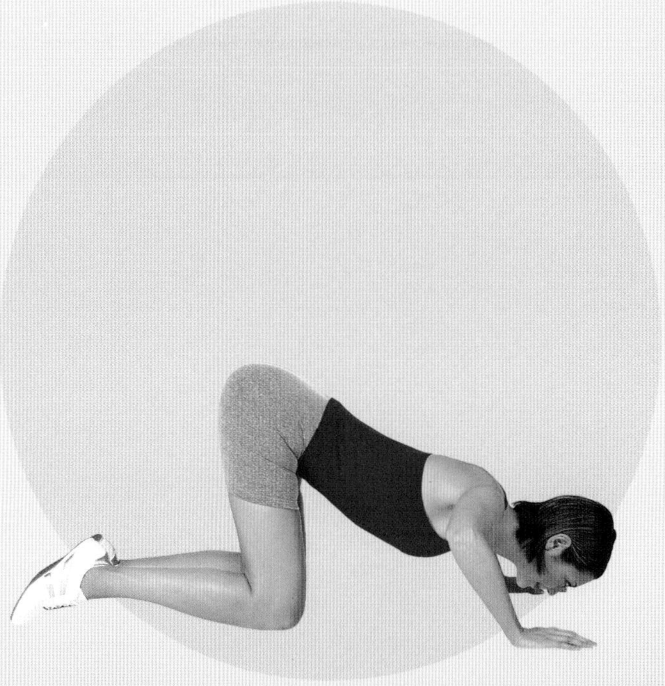

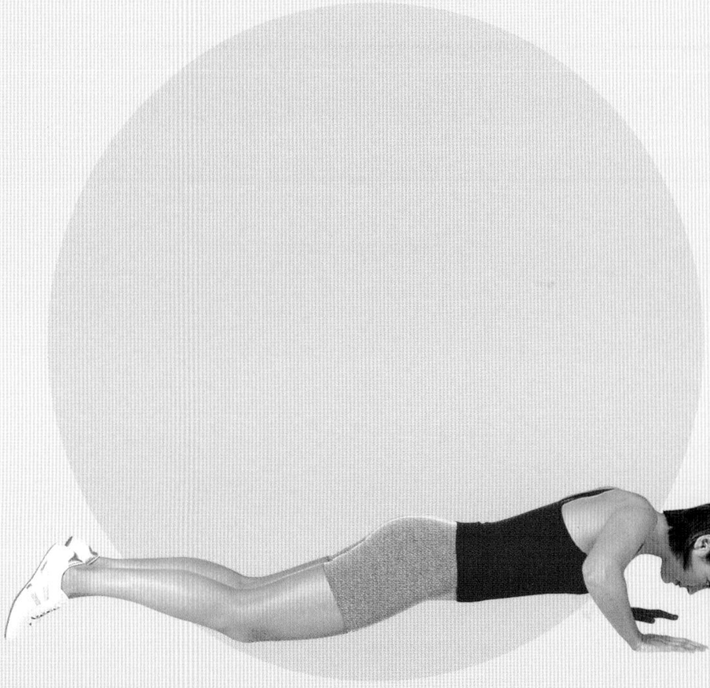

PROBLEM: **I can lower myself down but I can't lift my body back up.**

SOLUTION: **Start on all fours, but place your hands slightly wider than shoulder-width apart. Keep your hips lined up over your knees as you lower your chest toward the floor. In this position you are working with less body weight.**

PROBLEM: **I tend to sag in the middle when I do a full press up.**

SOLUTION: **Start in the extended, full Press-up position. Place your knees on the floor, hip-distance apart. Ensure that you keep your hips straight as you lower your chest toward the floor. Don't forget to switch on your core muscles.**

Back extension (arms by side)

SOLUTIONS

Problems with this exercise can arise from weakness in the mid or lower back and stiffness in the joints of the spine. This can result in back pain. Try to maintain a good breathing rhythm and avoid holding your breath as you lift your chest and hold the lift.

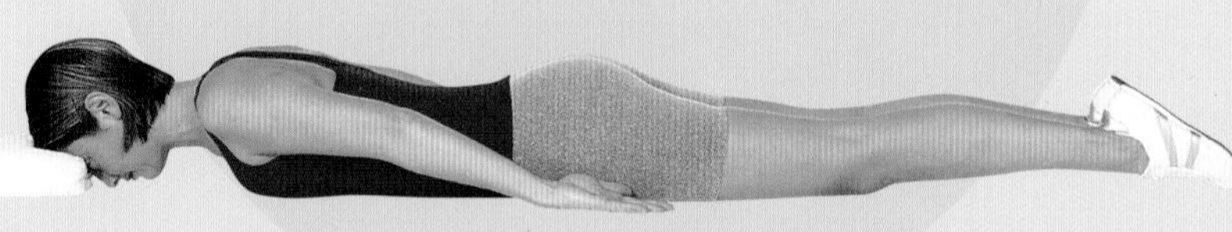

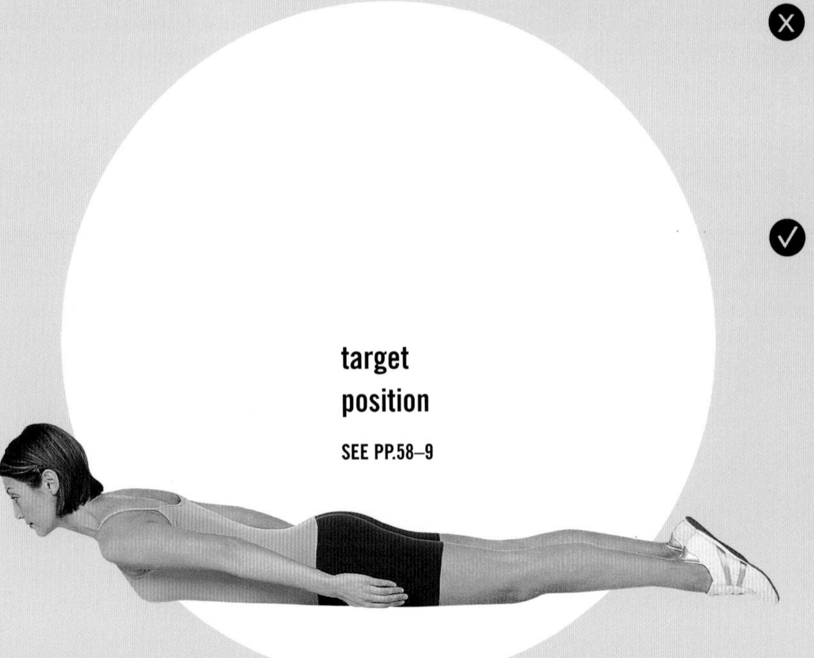

target position

SEE PP.58–9

PROBLEM: **My shoulders and shoulder blades keep rising up toward my ears.**

SOLUTION: **Start with your shoulders relaxed as you lie on your stomach, roll your shoulders back and think of pulling your shoulder blades down your back toward your waist or into the back pockets of a pair of jeans.**

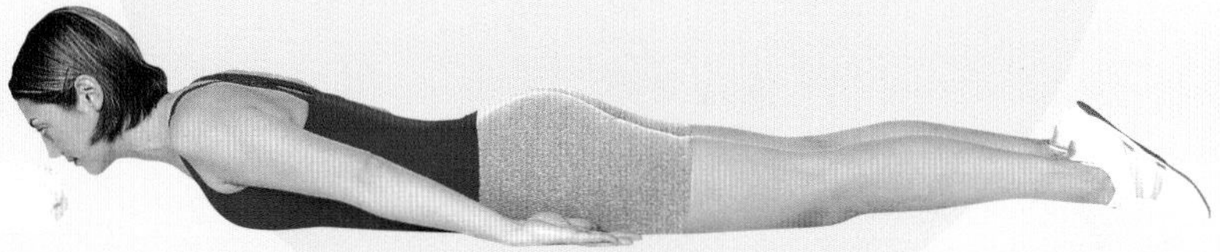

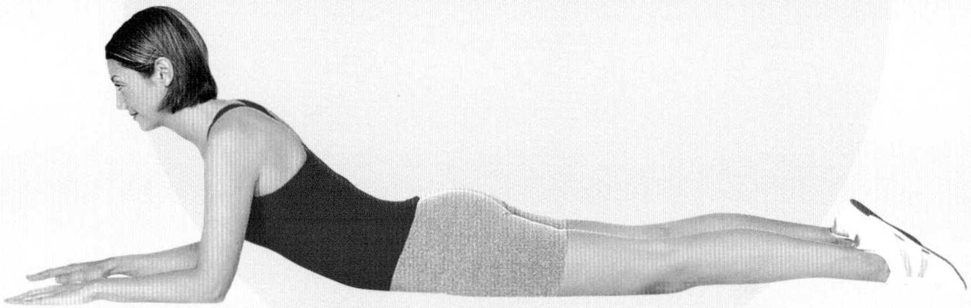

PROBLEM: **I would like to make the shoulder roll a little bit more taxing.**

SOLUTION: **As you roll your shoulders and shoulder blades back and down, lift your head ½ inch (1cm) off the towel, hold for 4 seconds and release. Keep the backs of your hands on the floor, and your neck long.**

PROBLEM: **I have a weak lower back.**

SOLUTION: **Raise yourself up onto your forearms (with the palms of your hands flat on the floor) so that your forearms take some of your body weight and help support your upper body as you work your lower back. As you get stronger put more weight onto your hands and ease your elbows off the floor.**

Hamstring curls (on all fours)

SOLUTION

Some of the elements of this position are wrist, arm and shoulder joint strength. A common complaint is that the wrists start to hurt the longer the position is held. The solution addresses weak wrists and can also be used by anyone suffering from carpal tunnel syndrome.

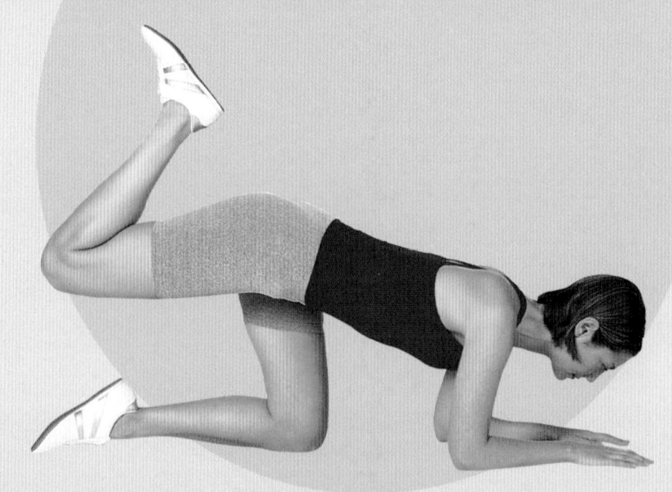

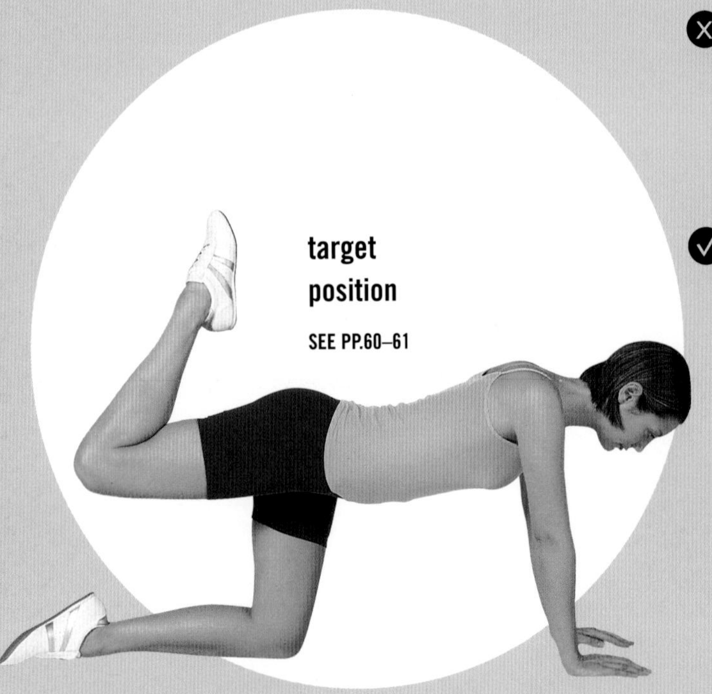

target position

SEE PP.60–61

PROBLEM: **My wrists start to hurt and then I can't complete all the repetitions.**

SOLUTION: **Place your forearms on the floor with your elbows under your shoulders to take the stress off your wrists. However, try to do some repetitions on your hands so that your wrists will eventually get stronger.**

Modified "T" stand

SOLUTION

This exercise may be difficult at first because balance is required in a side-lying position and there is very little of the body's surface in contact with the floor. In addition, the supporting shoulder joint takes a good amount of the body weight and it may not be used to this amount of stress.

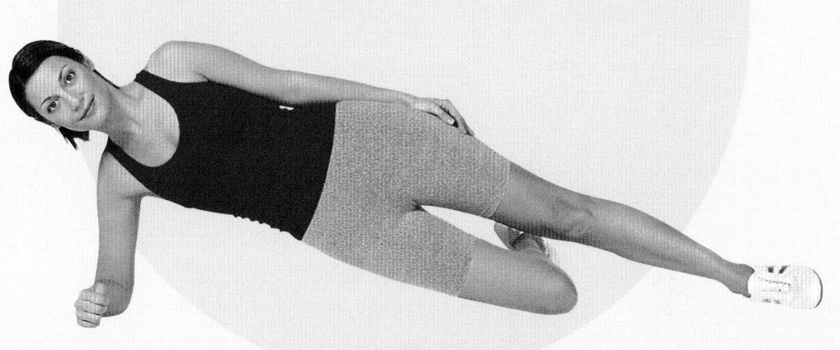

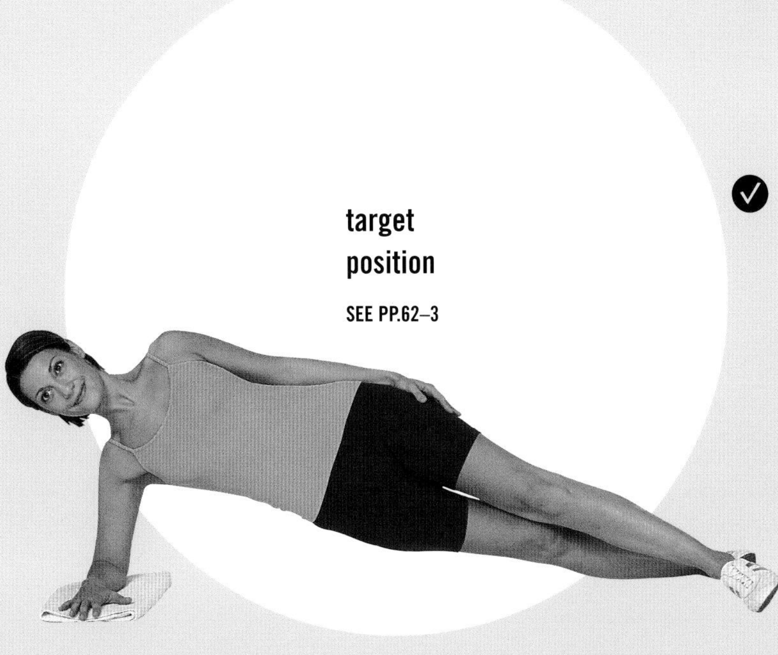

target position

SEE PP.62–3

PROBLEM: **I can't take that amount of weight through my forearm and shoulder.**

SOLUTION: **Bend your lower leg so that your knee is on the floor (directly under the knee of your top leg) and your lower leg is bent behind you. Your shoulder will then be supporting less body weight. Remember to keep your body in a straight line from ear to ankle**

Bridge

SOLUTIONS

The Bridge position can be hard to hold if your core muscles are weak or not properly engaged. It can also be difficult to smoothly roll up into the bridge if the lower back is stiff and has lost some of its mobility. If you find that you can't keep your hips up, try the Prone Leg Lift solution (p.91) to strengthen your gluteals.

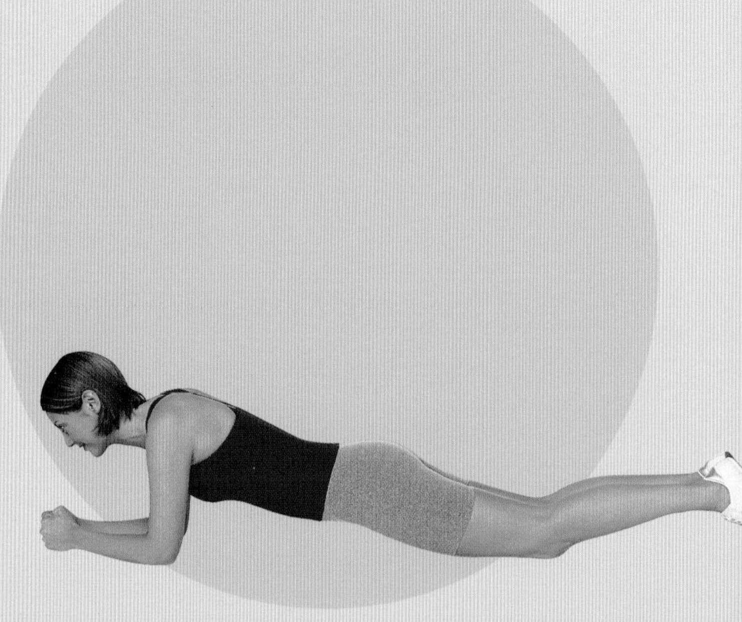

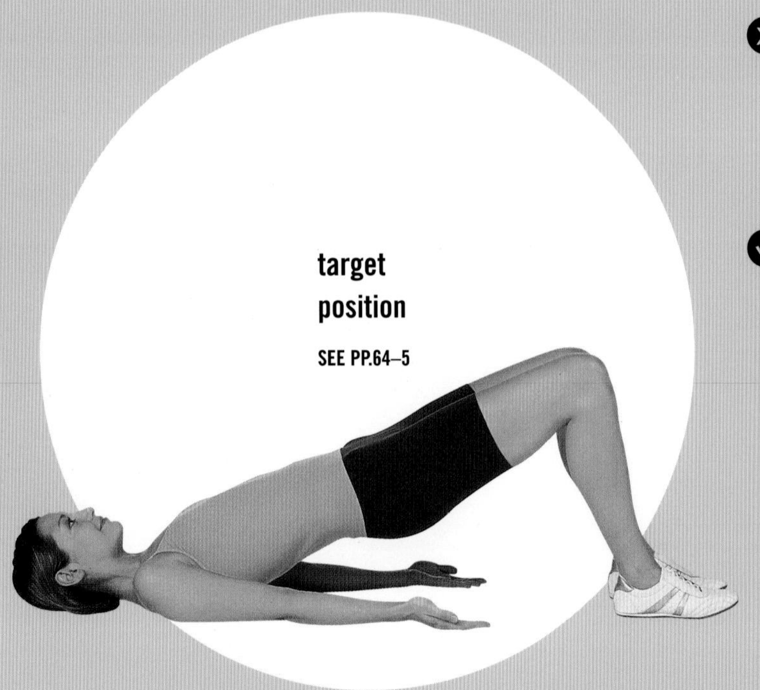

target position

SEE PP.64–5

PROBLEM: **I start to sag in the middle as I am trying to hold the position.**

SOLUTION: **Support yourself on your forearms and knees. Position your body so that your ears, shoulders, hips and knees are in a diagonal line. Breathe naturally as you hold the position for 10 to 20 seconds, then release. Repeat 5 times. This will strengthen the core muscles including the lower back.**

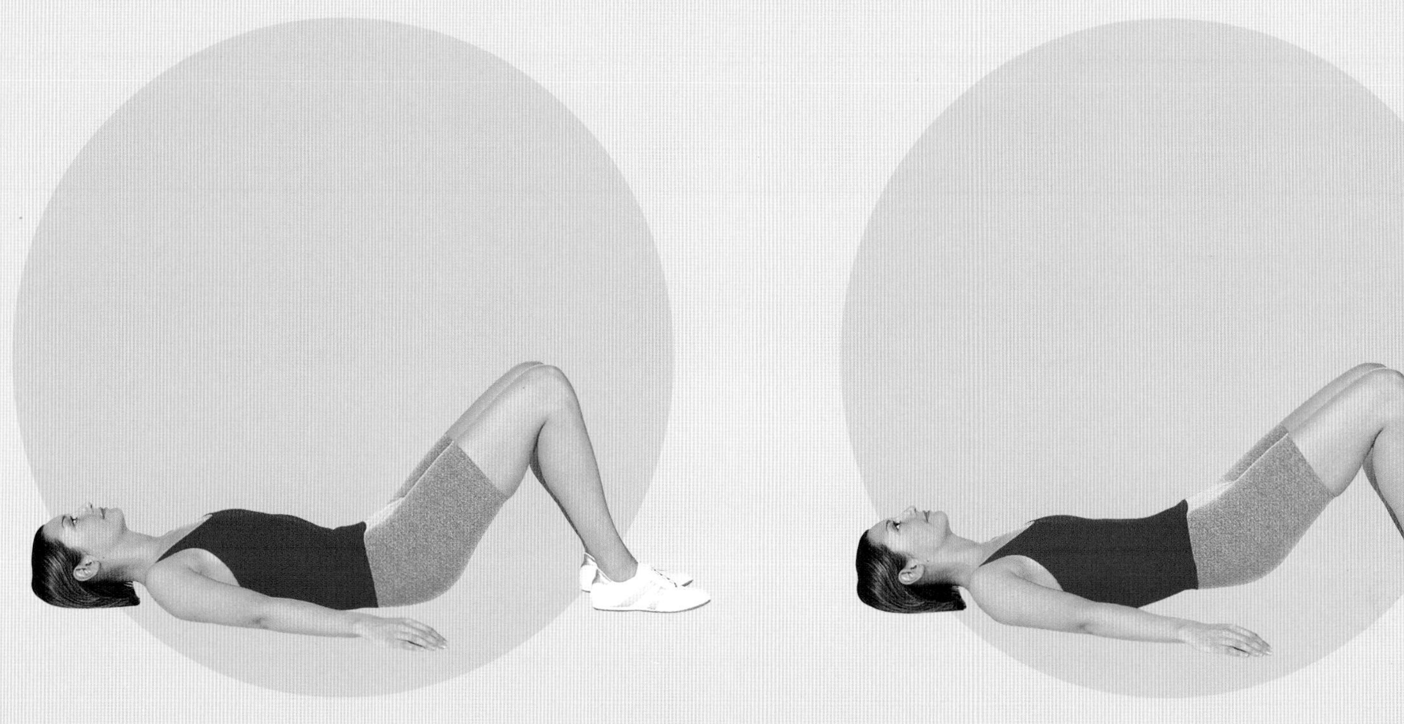

PROBLEM: **It feels as if I lift the whole of my lower back off the floor. I can't seem to work through each joint.**

SOLUTION: **Lie on the floor in the start position for the Bridge. Tilt your pelvis backward and press your lower back into the floor as you lift your bottom just off the floor. Release by rolling the lower spine back onto the floor and bringing your pelvis back into a neutral position.**

PROBLEM: **My hamstrings always start to cramp when I am in the Bridge position.**

SOLUTION: **This is a common occurrence in over-active, tense hamstrings. Doing a Hamstring and Hip Flexor Stretch (pp.66–7) before you do the Bridge will relax these muscles, encouraging the gluteals to work better in holding the hips up and reducing the risk of hamstring cramp. Also try positioning your feet further away from your bottom.**

Lying hamstring with calf and hip flexor stretch

SOLUTION

As this is a combination stretch it places a lot of functional demands on the whole body in terms of strength and flexibility. If necessary, the stretch can be sectioned and you can choose to do a specific part of the stretch.

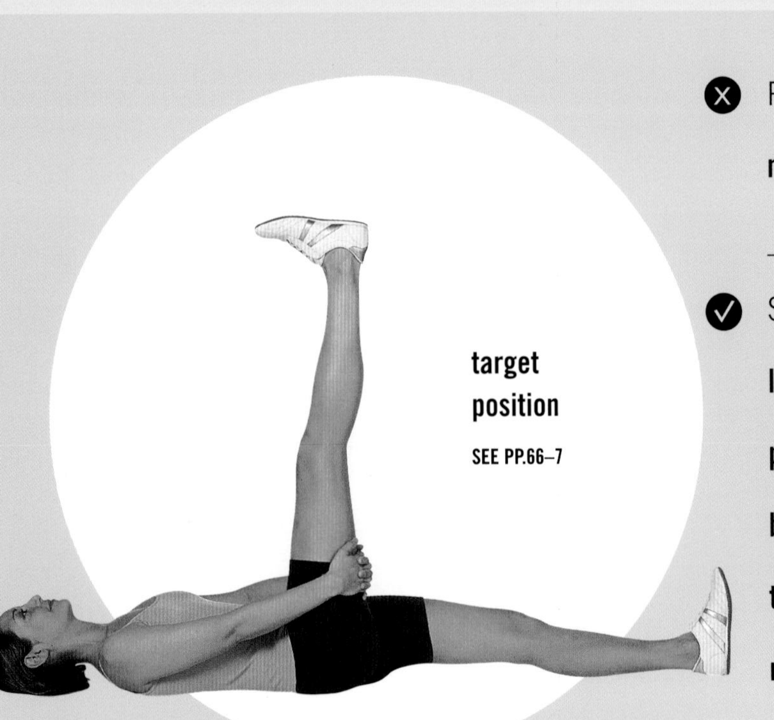

target position
SEE PP.66–7

PROBLEM: **This combination stretch hurts my lower back.**

SOLUTION: **Bend the knee of the second leg and place your foot on the floor. This position will provide more support for your back, however, it does mean that you will lose the hip flexor stretch. Check that your hips do not lift off the floor.**

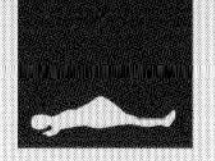

Gluts and chest stretch

VARIATION

This stretch is easily achievable by most people and does not require a solution. I have given a variation that will target the same main muscle groups. The original position also targets the muscles that cause the hip to turn out, whereas this variation does not.

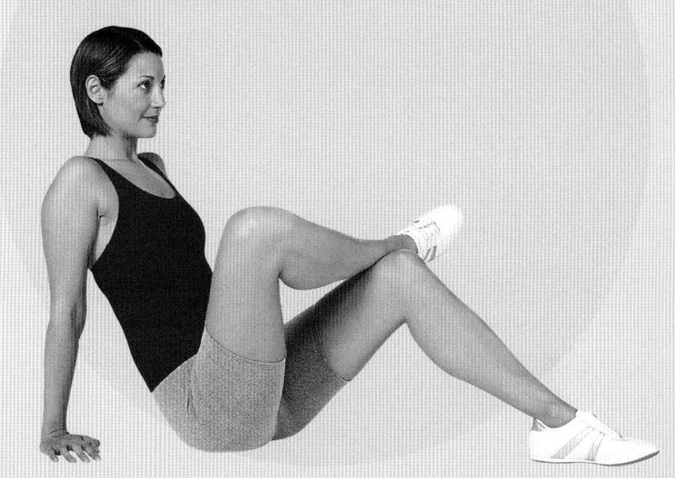

PROBLEM: **I would like to be able to target the same muscle groups from a seated position.**

SOLUTION: **Sit on the floor. Bend your right knee and place your right foot on your left thigh. Keeping your left heel on the floor, draw your left thigh toward your chest. Place your hands behind you to support yourself and roll the shoulders back to open your chest.**

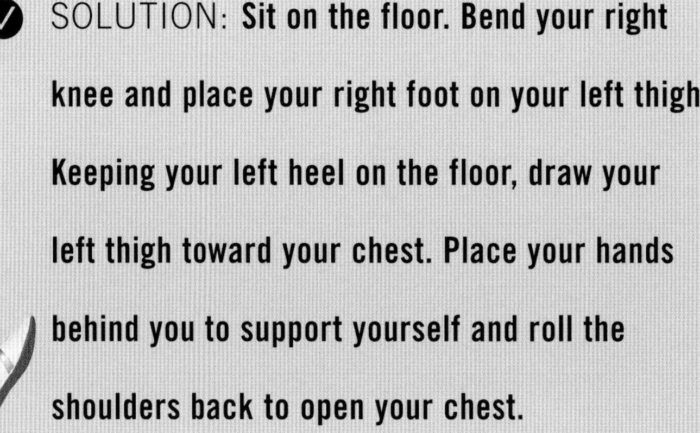

target position

SEE PP.68–9

Side-lying quad with hip flexor stretch

SOLUTION

This is a position that challenges stabilization while you stretch. The body has to balance on a relatively small amount of body surface area. The solution allows the body to be fully supported by the floor as the stretch takes place.

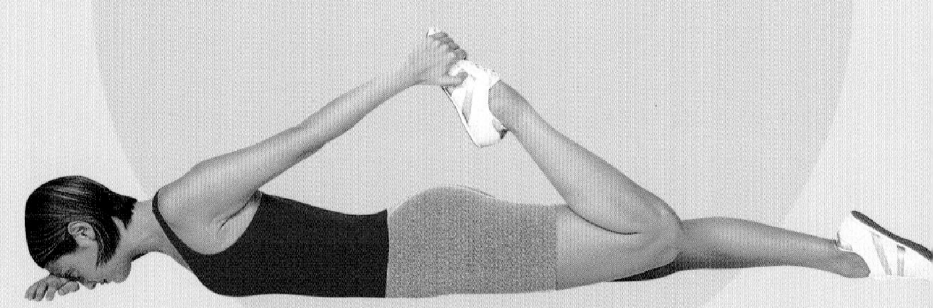

target position

SEE PP.70–71

PROBLEM: **I find it difficult to hold this position and focus on the stretch.**

SOLUTION: **Lie on your stomach to provide a more stable position. Lift your heel toward your bottom, holding on to your ankle or foot with your hand. Gently lift your knee off the floor while pressing your hips into the floor.**

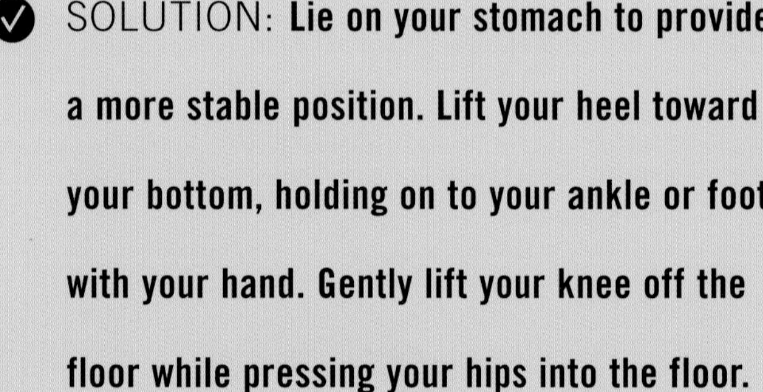

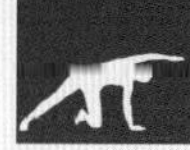

Lateral stretch

SOLUTION

This is a great stretch that has a real feel good factor. If it is not comfortable for you in the kneeling position because of discomfort in your knees and/or wrists try the suggested alternative.

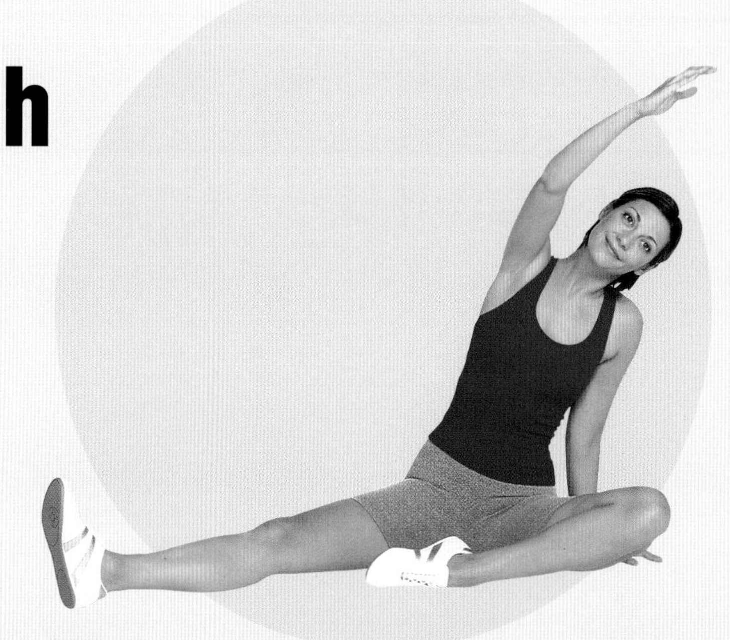

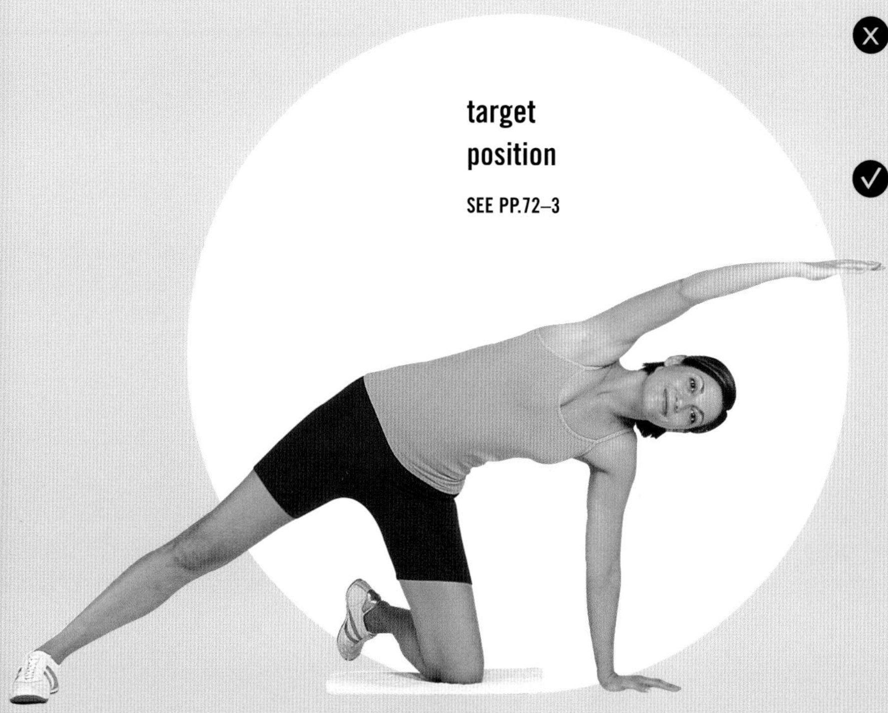

target position

SEE PP.72–3

PROBLEM: **It hurts my wrist and my knee.**

SOLUTION: **Sit on the floor with your legs crossed or in any position that is comfortable. Place your right hand on the floor and stretch your left arm overhead. Ensure your palm is facing the floor.**

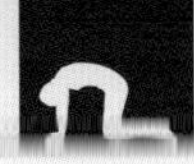

Cat stretch

SOLUTION

If doing this stretch on the floor causes a problem for joints, you won't get the full benefit from relaxing as you stretch. Tension tends to distract from the stretch physically and mentally.

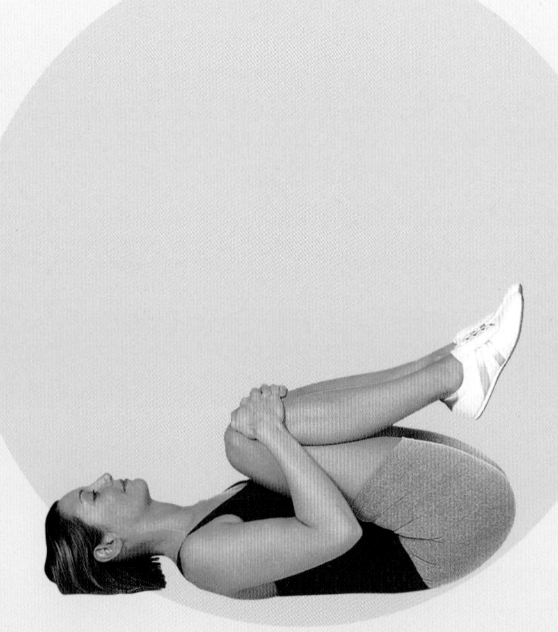

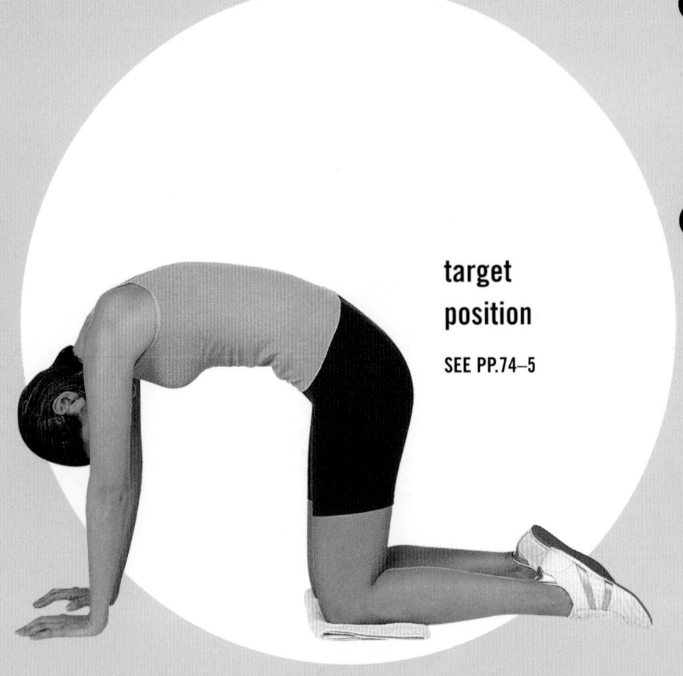

target position

SEE PP.74–5

PROBLEM: **This position causes discomfort in my knees and wrists.**

SOLUTION: **Lie on your back. Place your arms around your shins and pull your knees toward your chest. The back of your head should remain on the floor. Hold the position for 3 to 5 deep breaths. Release and repeat another 3 times.**

Easy Planning

– I DON'T HAVE TIME!

"I don't have time" is one of the most common reasons given for why we don't exercise. Ultimately, fitting exercise into our already busy lives comes down to skilled time management. Research indicates that the results of activity are cumulative and so our daily quota does not have to be completed in one session. If you can do shorter bursts of activity that add up to at least 30 minutes on most days (say, 3 x 10 minute-stints) health benefits will still be gained. The following table shows how you can modify your workout in Chapter 2 to fit the time you have. So, if you have 30 minutes to exercise, choose to do either the cardiovascular or the strength sections and alternate the days on which you do these. You should always do a warm-up before cardio-vascular activity, and cool down and stretch afterwards. Although you need to be warmed up for the strength moves, cooling down is not as essential if there has not been a big change in your breathing, body temperature etc. It is still important to stretch after a strength section as this allows time for your heart rate to come down.

WORKOUT COMPONENT	WORKOUT LENGTH (MINUTES)			
TOTAL TIME	30	30	45	60
Warm-up	5	5	7	8
Cardiovascular	12		12	18
Cool down	4		4	6
Strength		16	12	16
Flexibility	5	5	5	7
Relaxation	4	4	5	5

NOTE: In the cardiovascular section, 12 minutes equals 60 seconds for each exercise and the circuit is done twice. 18 minutes equals 90 seconds for each exercise and the circuit is done twice. In the strength section, if time is short, choose to do the Single Leg Squat one day and the Lunge the next time. You can also leave out the Prone Leg Lift, as the gluteals will get some work in the Hamstring Curl exercise.

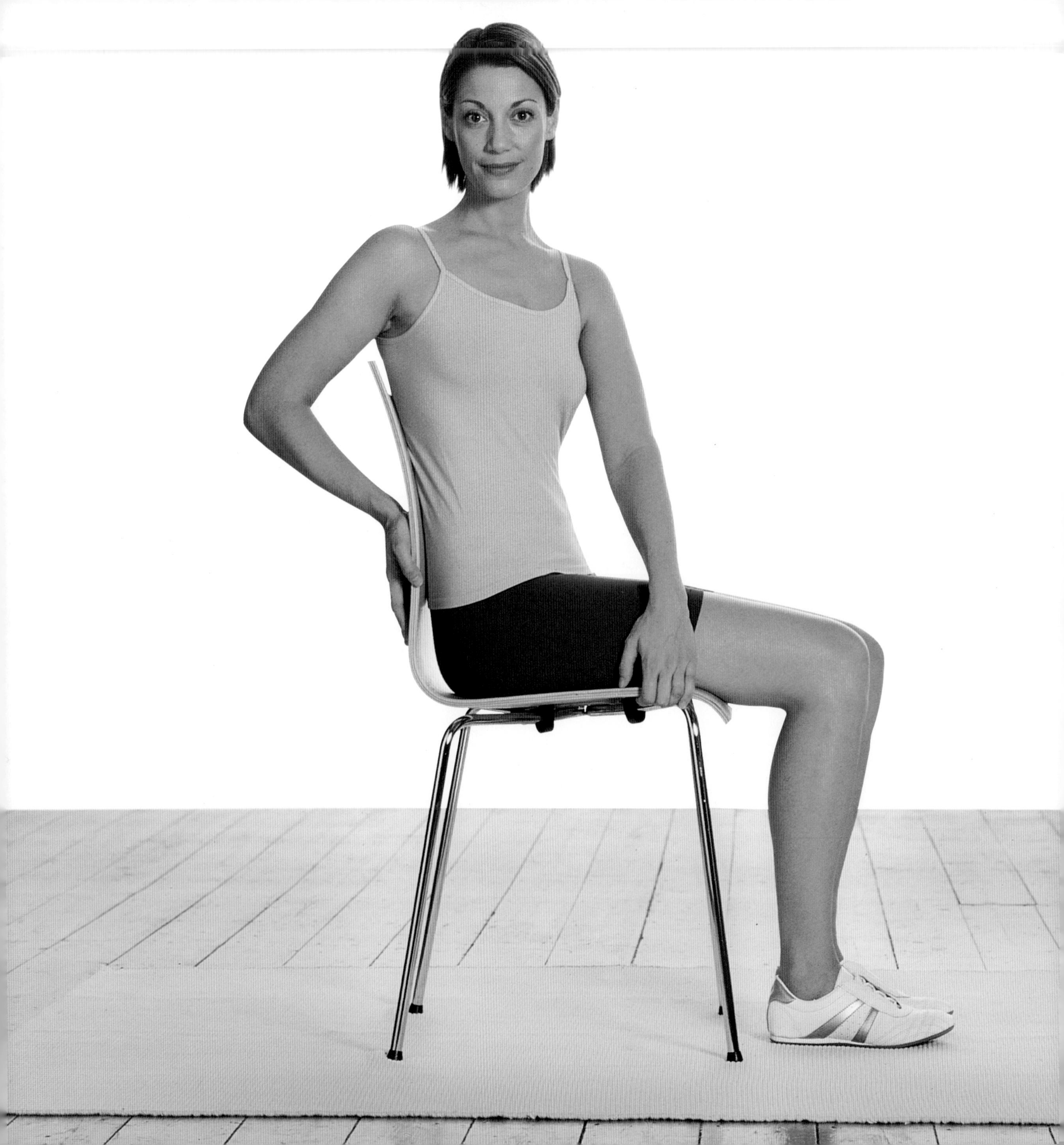

CHAPTER 4: Easy Cool-down

In the same way that a warm-up is essential to ensure that the transition from not exercising to exercising is smooth, and that the exercise experience itself is effective and safe, an active cool-down is also an important part of the workout.

This chapter explains why you should cool down and what the effect of cooling down is on the different body systems. I provide you with a cool-down sequence to follow that takes you smoothly and safely from exercise mode to a condition close to your pre-exercise state. You can also do the warm-up sequence in reverse as another cool-down option.

You should always follow cardiovascular activity with a cool-down. However, if you have chosen to do the strength section rather than the cardiovascular section, the cool-down is not essential because the changes in the body will not be as great. The strength sequence finishes on the floor, so the stretches can double as your cool-down.

Why cool down?

The objective of a cool-down is to gradually return the body to its pre-exercise state. Rhythmic movements of decreasing intensity, keeping the arms below shoulder level and performing activity that promotes the return of blood from the extremities to the heart, will all achieve this.

There are a number of physiological changes that should happen during the cool-down. The heart rate should decrease and return to normal or just above its resting rate. If you are relying on the Rate of Perceived Exertion scale (see p.78), you should aim to be at a 1 or 2 (hardly no effort–very, very easy).

As an exercise becomes more intense, your body will produce more waste products and by-products, such as lactic acid, which is thought to contribute to muscle soreness and stiffness. These acids accumulate in the blood. The cool-down ensures that the circulatory system keeps working hard enough to rid the body of most, if not all, the waste products and lactic acid, which should help reduce the incidence of soreness.

Stopping moving immediately after vigorous or intense exercise, especially when you have been standing, can cause blood to pool in the large muscles of your legs. If your legs have been doing a lot of work, a large percentage of the body's blood supply will be in that area, which means there is less blood available for your heart and brain. The reduced supply of blood to your brain can starve it of oxygen, resulting in dizziness and fainting. Remaining active, at a low level, assists the return of the blood to the heart and brain, so avoiding this type of situation.

Body temperature will lower as the activity decreases because the energy production system will not be generating as much heat as a by-product of producing energy. This heat is dissipated through the skin as perspiration. As the body temperature drops, the body no longer needs as much cooling and so the circulatory system stops taking as much blood to the surface of the skin.

The amount of blood within the muscles will also reduce. During the warm-up and cardiovascular/main exercises, the blood supply to the muscles increases so that the blood can transport essential oxygen and nutrients to the cells, which are then used in the energy-making process. As the body cools down, this process slows down and the blood supply can return to its normal job of carrying oxygen and nutrients to internal organs, such as the liver and digestive system.

Breathing rate, which will have increased with the increase in exercise intensity, will drop during the cool-down. You should aim for a level of activity that you can very easily maintain without any sign of breathlessness. At this level, you should be able to speak 4 or 5 words without having to take a breath.

If the exercise segment has been very vigorous and breathing rate has increased a great amount, almost to where you cannot catch your breath, which might happen in the cardiovascular section, you may have been working anaerobically. Anaerobic training is cardiovascular exercise that uses a different energy system from aerobic training. Whereas aerobic training uses oxygen in the production of energy, anaerobic training does not.

Breathing demands become higher and harder as you edge up the intensity ladder and move from the aerobic to the anaerobic system. One way to encourage your breathing to return to a normal rate after vigorous activity is to focus on making your out-breath longer than your in-breath. If your in-breath takes 4 to 5 seconds, try and slow your out-breath so that it takes 8 to 10 seconds. This can assist in slowing down your breathing rate generally. You have to focus on your breath in order to do this effectively.

Focusing on your breathing in this way also has psychological implications. It allows you to switch your attention and concentration from external factors, such as your environment, and how you have been doing the exercises, to more internally-centered elements, such as how well you are doing and how you feel. The cool-down gives you time to assess how you did in the cardiovascular/main section. You can think about whether you worked at an appropriate level, too hard or not hard enough and you can set your target for next time.

If you are including all the components of the Easy Fitness workout in your session, the cool-down allows you to mentally ease out of the cardiovascular section and prepare for the strength section. This part of the workout will be demanding in a different way and may require a change of attitude or thinking strategy. If you are great at cardiovascular exercise but not so good at strength moves, the resistance section may be more challenging for you and demand greater focus. The reverse may be true, perhaps you are muscularly strong but weak in endurance activities. The cool-down is an ideal opportunity to make any required or desired mind change.

Physical activity can result in improved self-esteem and self-awareness. It can make you more outgoing because you feel better about yourself and are more positive about how others will see/accept you. The cool-down allows time to acknowledge these feelings of well-being, of having done and achieved something, in having invested time in yourself that positively affects your mental attitude about yourself and your life in general. Try to carry this positive attitude into the strength and flexibility sections, as well as your relaxation session and your approach toward everyday life.

Cool-down sequence

In order for the cool-down to be gradual, sufficient time must be allocated within the session. 5 to 10 minutes is recommended. Cooling down is primarily achieved through decreasing the intensity of exercises through smaller range of movement. However, dynamic stretching, where the muscle is actively taken through its full range of movement, can be included toward the end of your cool-down. If your workout includes some resistance work, it is also a good idea to statically stretch out the muscles that you are going to work next.

The exercises in the sequence work to cool down the whole body at once. The movements involve both the upper and lower body, but the arms should stay at or below shoulder level, as when the arms are raised above the head for any length of time, the heart has to work harder to pump blood up to the hands.

The Side Step with Lateral Raise serves to keep the body moving, but at a lower level of intensity than is maintained in the main section. The use of the large leg muscles helps with venous blood return (return of blood to the heart and brain), and the arms give some balance to the movement.

The Heel Digs with Hand Shakes are "on the spot", so that activity of the whole body is reduced, but there is still movement of specific parts. Shaking out the hands and arms is good for releasing any tension that might be held in the hands, arms, shoulders or neck.

Rear Lunges are included in this section as an orientation for the Lunges to follow in the strength section. They open out the front of the hips that have been in a flexed or bent position for a lot of the cardiovascular work. The Punches are done with open fingers to ensure tension does not return to the arms and hands. They dynamically lengthen the latissimus dorsi muscles located under the shoulder blades.

Lastly, the Marches bring the movement discipline down to a base line, in the same way that walking is a foundational movement. This is a good opportunity to take 3 or 4 deep breaths to calm the body and the mind. The arm circles should help to open out the lungs on the inhale and exhale of breath. These breaths serve to bring this section of the workout to a close and should help you refocus and re-energize for the coming strength or flexibility section.

Take the opportunity to have a drink of water at the end of the cool-down section. Fluid replacement is vital to performance and dehydration can cause headaches, dizziness and disorientation. Drink in sips rather than gulps and have water that is room temperature or is slightly chilled rather than very cold water. You should ensure that you drink throughout the workout too, so have a bottle of water handy. When you stop for a drink, don't stop moving but keep marching or side stepping to keep blood circulation going.

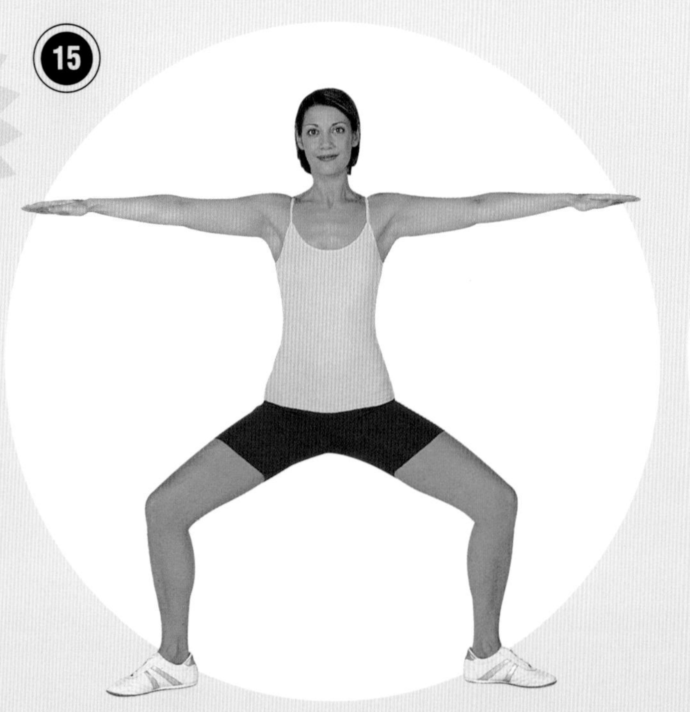

Side step with lateral raise

Take 2 big side steps to your right and then 2 steps back to your left. As you step out, lift your arms out to the side to shoulder height. When you step your feet together, your arms should cross in front of your body. After 16 repetitions, rest your hands on your hips and do 8 double side steps without using your arms. Then make your steps smaller and more comfortable for another 8 repetitions.

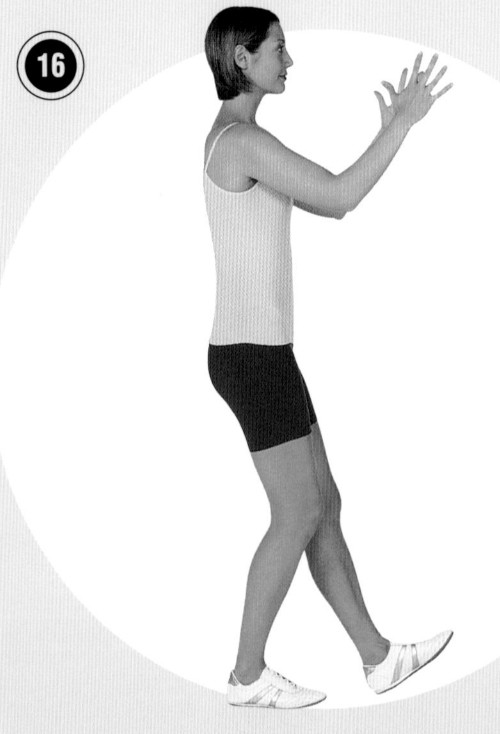

Heel digs with hand shakes

Stand tall with your feet hip-distance apart and facing forward. Step your right foot forward and touch the floor with your heel. Your toes should be lifted. Replace your right foot and do the same with your left foot. As you heel dig, raise your hands to chest height and shake out your wrists and fingers. As your foot steps back in place, shake your wrists and fingers by your side. Do 20 repetitions.

17

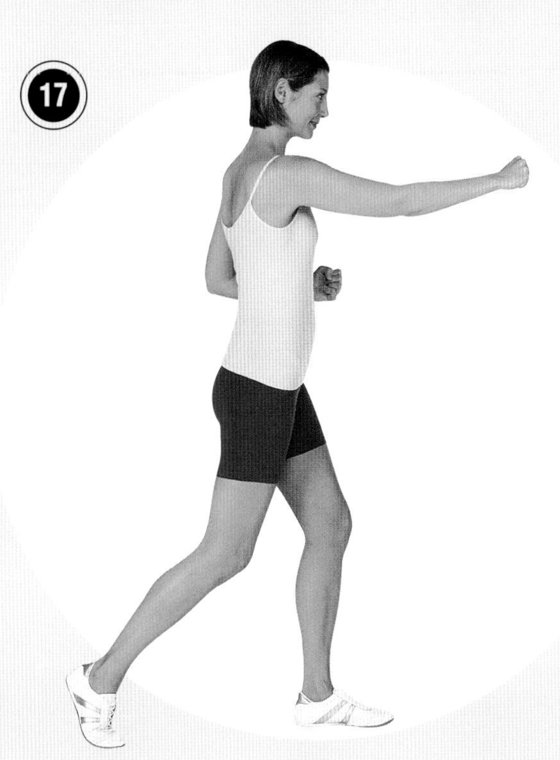

18

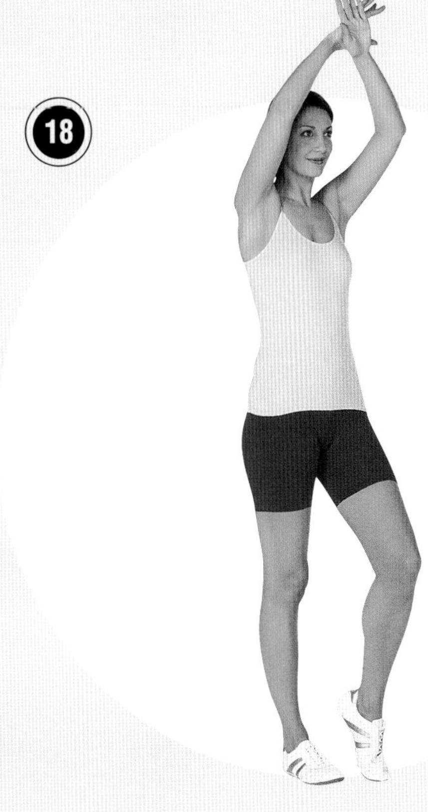

Rear lunge with easy punch

Take your right foot behind you and tap the floor with your toes. Replace this foot and do the same with your left foot. As your right foot taps back, punch forward with your right arm and vice versa. Repeat 8 times with each leg. Then change so that you punch with your left arm as you tap back with your right leg. Do 8 repetitions with each leg. Keep your fists loose to avoid a build up of tension in neck and arms.

Walk and march

This is easy! Walk around in the space available, swinging your arms by your side. Focus on your breathing. This should now be returning to a normal rate. Once you feel your breathing is back to normal or almost there, march on the spot and take 3 or 4 focused breaths. Take your arms out to the side and overhead as you breathe in. Replace your arms by your side as you breathe out.

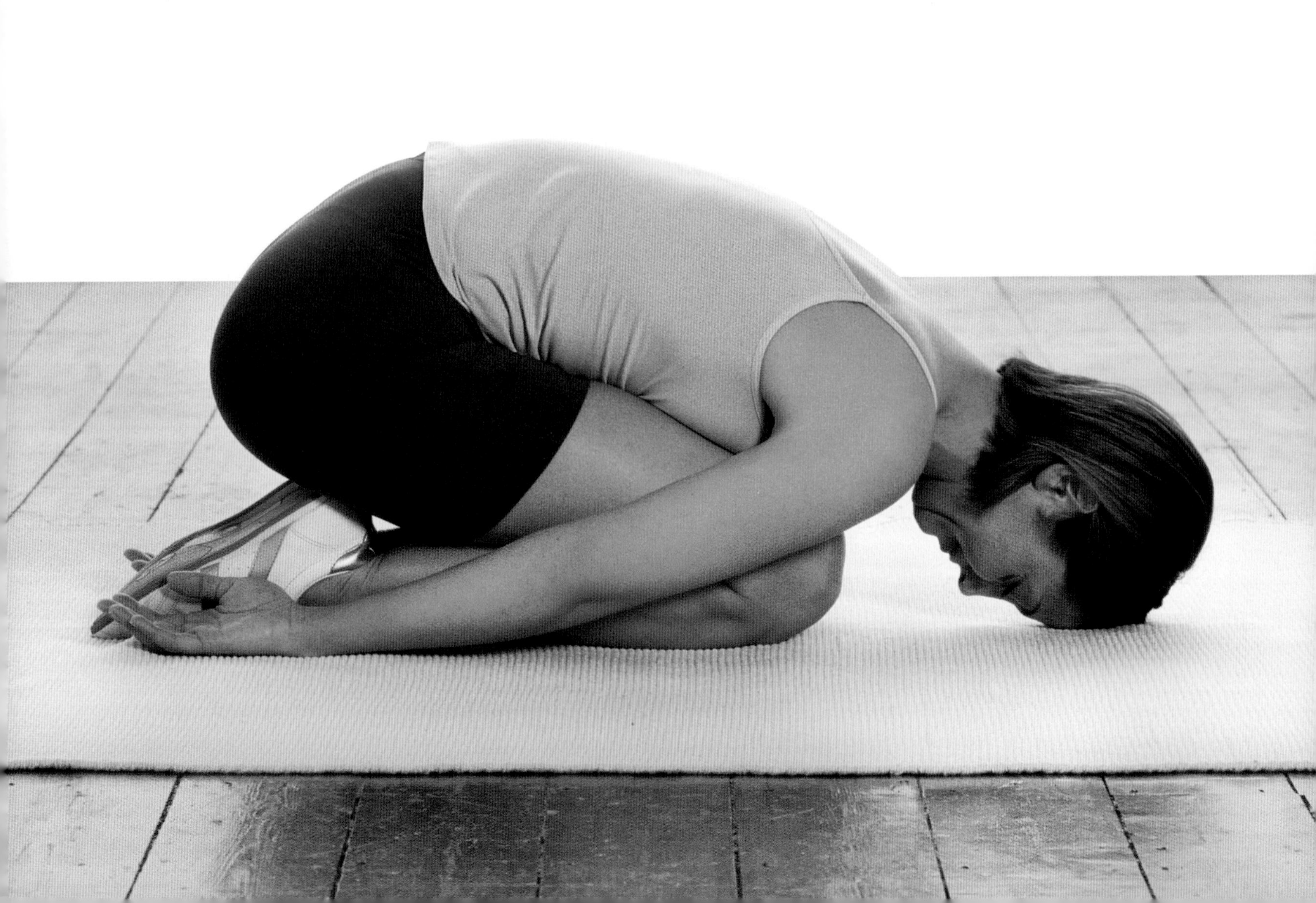

CHAPTER 5: Easy Relaxation

Relaxation has an important role to play in giving balance to our lives. Think of any machine that is constantly on the go. It will burn itself out more quickly than a machine that has "down time". The body is an intricate and complex mechanism that needs rest and relaxation to function properly on both a mental and physical level. If we consider that sleep is not always restful, and that lack of sleep can affect our immune system, the ability and opportunity to relax while at rest is crucial to general health and well-being.

This chapter starts by looking at how exercise releases stress and prepares the body for relaxation. We look at the importance of making time for relaxation and creating a particular place to relax, as well as techniques to enable you to relax in stressful situations. I then take you through 2 relaxation postures and a breathing exercise to assist the process of calming and re-energizing the mind and the body.

Relaxation and fitness

The body has a natural cycle in the same way that nature has the cycle we interpret as the seasons. We can look at the daily routine of the body in terms of seasons. Spring is the waking up to a new day. Summer is when nature is at its busiest and full of energy. It is the time for going out to work, doing chores and daily activities; being up and active. Late summer is the afternoon when the body starts to slow down and energy levels are generally lower. Autumn is the return home after your day. A time to relax and shed the stresses of the day in preparation for the closing down phase of sleep. Winter is sleep, a time for rest and rejuvenation. The body needs this time to recharge.

Relaxation is part of a natural balance and a shift in that balance will affect our general well-being. If the mind is not relaxed, quality of sleep can be adversely affected, and we may suffer loss of appetite or we may turn to stress eating. If we are not physically relaxed we can be quite restless, use up a lot of energy and feel constantly tired.

We need to be able to unwind and relax after a stressful day or event. And we sometimes need to be able to relax while in a stressful situation. The stress that we find hard to cope with is not always "bad" stress. It may simply be stress caused by a lot of mental and/or physical demands being made on the body over a period of time. Take the image of unwinding. If you wind up something mechanical it usually has a chance to unwind over time. If that something were to remain constantly wound up, and therefore under tension, it would eventually breakdown or stop working. The human body is the same.

We need to acknowledge that stress does not necessarily get released because we go into relaxation mode. Certain personality types can find it hard to relax. People with stressful jobs or in stressful situations may not be able to just "switch off". If you are one of these people, a form of activity, such as a boxing class, a run, a power walk or a yoga session, may be a necessary prerequisite to, or a essential part of, your relaxation session. Activity is "time out" for the mind, as it enables you to focus on something other than the issues that are foremost in the mind or it can allow time for focused thinking that helps clarify issues and may result in a solution.

Activity can aid the release of frustration, anxiety and stress, as well as muscular tension. In stressful situations the body releases fuels and hormones in what it recognizes as a primitive "fight or flight" response. However, in most stressful situations today, it is inappropriate to fight or flee! And so the fuels and hormones remain in the blood stream and can become harmful to the body. Activity allows the body to use up these fuels and hormones, enabling us to better relax.

A time and a place

We should be able to find 10 to 15 minutes in which to relax every day, even if we are very busy. The ideal time to relax is toward the end of the day to aid restful sleep, but it is also important to be able to relax at any other necessary or desirable time during the day.

If you have the opportunity to relax in a favourite place, think about where best suits. It could be a spare room, your bedroom, the bathroom or any other room that makes you feel calm. Try to create an environment that will aid your mental and physical relaxation. The room should be uncluttered and free of distracting objects. Use colours and lighting to establish a warm and calm ambience. Consider what position you want to relax in, noting that this may change from day to day. The furniture and fittings in your chosen area should allow you to sit, kneel or lie comfortably. Ensure the space is warm enough but not overly hot and remember to wear comfortable clothing.

Although relaxation is often associated with a specific time of day or a particular place, it is good to cultivate the ability to relax any time and anywhere. That way whenever you are faced with a stressful situation, you will be better equipped to deal with the stress and tension. For example, you may need to relax at work because you feel challenged by the workload or a colleague; you may be travelling in between meetings and need a few minutes to relax and compose yourself on the train; or you may have a group of loudly playing children in the house and need a few minutes to yourself to be able to cope for the next hour.

In any such situation you should have a relaxation strategy to fit your circumstances. So, if you are at home you might practise a relaxation posture (p.122–3) or if you are at your desk you might take five minutes to do a seated breathing exercise (p.124–5). Train yourself in that strategy as you would with any other skill. The more you practise, the easier it will be for you to enter a state of relaxation.

If you find it difficult to relax in a certain situation, there are different tools you can use to trigger relaxation. You could use a breathing technique or a body position, or you might choose a smell, a texture or an object, or something else that activates a sense of calm.

As the day draws to a close, try to avoid stimulation such as television, coffee, alcohol, food, using the computer or telephone, etc.

Different people relax in different ways, so experiment to find a few ways that suit you. Take a hot bath or shower; meditate or just sit quietly; light candles; burn incense; play relaxing music; use essential oils such as lavender in your bath, on your pillow or on your night clothes; have a massage; do a stretch, yoga or Tai Chi routine; or read a book. The key is to choose a way to relax that meets your mental, physical and spiritual needs at any particular time, in any particular place.

Relaxation postures

The purpose of relaxation is to help restore equilibrium and reduce, if not release, physical and mental tension. Body position is a very important contributing factor to the success of a relaxation session. If a position is unbalanced in any way – if it adversely affects your breathing, makes you feel insecure or uncomfortable – this will become a distraction that affects your ability to relax in part or completely.

I have chosen two floor postures here because lying positions, as opposed to sitting ones, allow the body full support from the floor. This means that your muscles can relax from their usual state of assisting posture and/or movement and any physical tension is greatly reduced as a result.

The Corpse Pose, or lying straight out on the floor, is a great position for just letting go and allowing the floor to take your weight. Your breathing should be easy and free. When fully relaxed some people will naturally want to turn their head to one

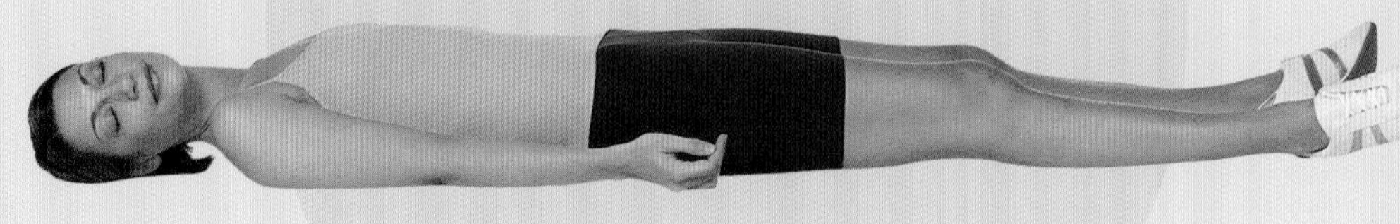

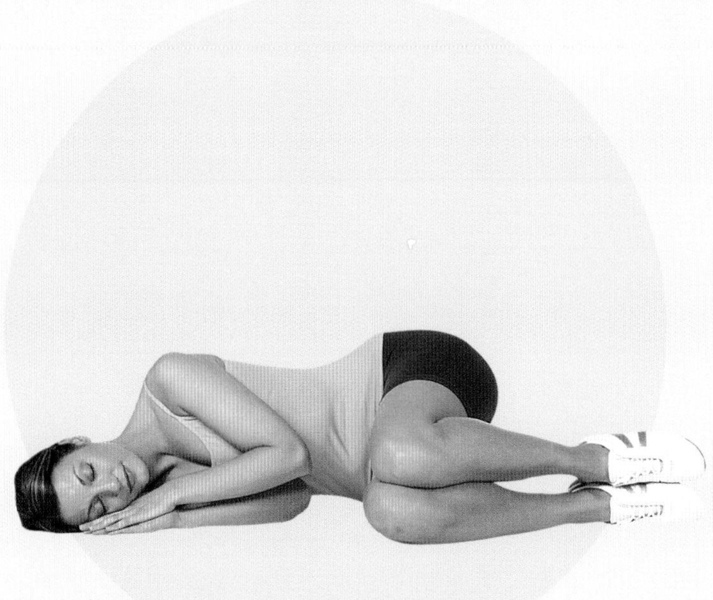

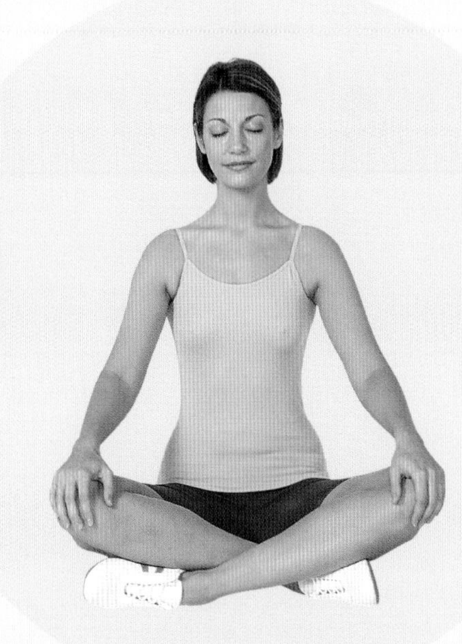

side or the other because holding the head aligned uses muscles and creates tension. It is safe to do this. If you experience any discomfort in your lower back in this position, bending your knees and placing your feet flat on the floor or placing a rolled-up towel under your lower back or knees will give your back a little more support and should make you comfortable.

Alternatively, you can turn onto your side and take up the Foetal Position. This is a particularly natural and comfortable position to adopt. The feelings and emotions attached to it are closely related to feeling protected, warm and secure in the womb and it is a position many people assume when they sleep. Even though it is a fairly "closed" position, your breathing should not be adversely affected as you will be calm and settled.

You may find it just as easy to relax in a seated position and you can adopt this as your relaxation stance if you would prefer to do so.

Relaxing breath

Breathing correctly and focusing on your breath is a great way to aid relaxation.

The ability to relax is not only affected by external factors that cause stress, it is also dependant on your personality. Often, people who are very dynamic, competitive and demanding of themselves and others, who like to be doing lots of things at the same time and seem to thrive on stress, tend to find it hard to be quiet and still if their minds have nothing to concentrate on. If you find it difficult to relax, you should find breathing exercises especially useful. Concentrating on your breath can give you the focus you need to reach some level of relaxation and help you to enjoy being in a relaxed state, too.

When we are stressed or anxious our breathing becomes shallow and fast and our heart rate and blood pressure rise. The cardiorespiratory system is one body system that we can take steps to control. We can manipulate our breathing to calm ourselves. Focused breathing can slow your breathing rate and your heart rate, lower blood pressure and warm up your body.

Breathing is also of symbolic importance. It can be empowering to acknowledge our breath as a life giving force that we cannot exist without. Try the following breathing exercise that can be done any time and anywhere.

Sit or lie on the floor and close your eyes. Place one or both hands lightly on your stomach. Focus on your in-breath and your out-breath and ensure that your position does not restrict or hinder your breathing. Become aware of the depth and pace of your breathing without changing either. Try to breathe from deep down in your abdomen rather than from the upper part of your chest. As you breathe in, your stomach should expand. As you breathe out, your stomach flattens.

Acknowledge that each in-breath brings with it energy and vitality. Each out-breath takes with it something that you want to rid your body of, be it tiredness, frustration, anxiety, etc. This is an opportunity to let go of some, if not all, of those stresses that we collect and carry around through the day.

If, as you sit or lie on the floor, thoughts come into your mind, avoid latching on to them. Let them pass for the moment. Usually, if they are important, they will return later. Turn your attention back to your breath. If you find it difficult to remain focused, think of being calm and energized. Try to recall a time in the past when you have been in that state and picture yourself in those circumstances once more. Take a few minutes to reconnect with those resources and allow the feeling of what it was like to be calm and energized to stay with you once you are ready to open your eyes. Allow yourself a few moments to acclimatize before you slowly ease yourself to your feet and start moving again.

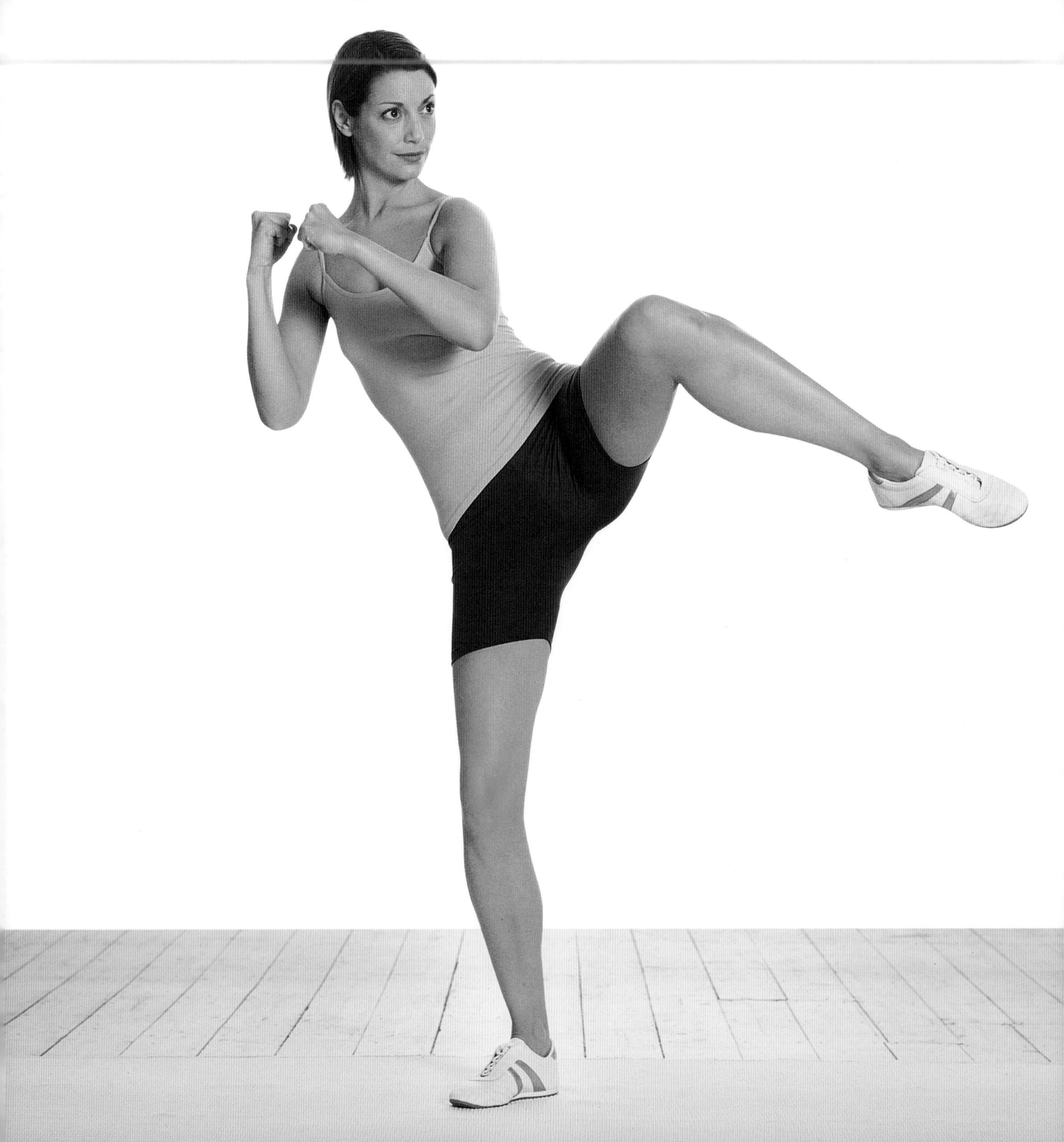

CHAPTER 6: Easy Fitness for Easy Sports

This chapter looks at how being fit can help your sport and how your training should be structured to ensure you perform well in, and get the most from, your chosen activity. The chapter is divided into five sporting areas: running, golf, racquet sports, ball sports, and combat sports. For each area I outline how the exercises detailed in the workout can help improve your fitness for that sport.

Running is a popular means of keeping fit, as well as a sport. All sports with an element of consistent running, such as soccer, basketball and even baseball, can benefit from the exercises described. I have included golf as it is an increasingly played, all-year-round sport. Racquet sports such as tennis, badminton and squash remain very popular. In the section on ball sports, I cover exercises for basketball and netball. Combat sports include martial arts and boxing, which are sports that have been practised in clubs and sports halls for decades and are now considered to be mainstream fitness activities.

Fitness first

Some people take up a sporting activity, such as squash or weekend soccer, as a leisure activity that will also get them fit. Most sports require a good base level of general fitness, aside from the specific skills of the game, in order for the sport to be played well. Assessing what the physical demands of the sport are will give you a good idea of what elements of fitness you need to cultivate before you start to play or train.

Unless your sport is static (for example, darts, archery, shooting), a base level of cardiovascular fitness is desirable. A good marker is whether you can do 20 minutes of continuous cardiovascular activity at a moderate pace, say 5–6 on the Rate of Perceived Exertion Scale discussed in Chapter 3 (see p.78).

Core strength is foundational to all sports, static and moving, for two reasons. First, the power of any movement should come from the core, and second, the core muscles need to be able to stabilize the torso and hold it strong as the limbs move. Core strength reduces the risk of injury around the back and shoulder girdle, helps stabilize the muscles of the legs, hip and pelvis and aids balance and coordination.

Strength and joint stability should be worked together because muscle strength aids joint stability. You need to be strong not just in the muscles that are being used but also in opposing muscles. Many sports cause muscle imbalance because one side or one section of the body is being used more than another, for example, a right-handed tennis or badminton player, or a cyclist who rides bent over for long periods, overstretching his/her back and constantly contracting through the abdominals. In order to minimize injury and maintain good posture, alignment and muscle balance, your training programme needs to combine exercises that make you better at the sport with exercises that address the stresses and imbalances placed on the body by the training and performance of the sport.

Flexibility and joint mobility should also be worked together. The more flexible you are, the more mobile you can be around a joint. Flexibility is the component worked on the least in sports (except for in dance or gymnastics), and yet it is just as important as the other elements in terms of lengthening and re-aligning muscles. For example, if we take the action of throwing a ball. Most people focus on the strength involved and train to develop strength in the arms and shoulders. Yet, they should also work on flexibility around the shoulder joint and the back, which comes into play as the arm is taken back in preparation for the throw, and as the throw is taken.

Regular general fitness training that covers all the fitness components discussed here will enable you to perform well in your sport and enhance your enjoyment of your game.

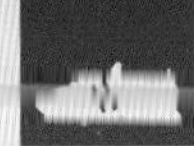

Easy fitness for running

The training for running is very specific and involves ... running, running and more running! You can work on your cardiovascular fitness in other sports, such as rowing or cycling, but because of the difference in the way the muscles are used for each of these activities, the muscular endurance gained in one activity does not easily cross over into the others.

The exercises for running will apply to all sports in which speed and distance affect performance, such as soccer and track events. For example, in soccer you would aim to develop speed to be able to reach the ball before your opponent or in a running event you may time yourself over a set distance to gauge improvement. Sprint-runs (pp.38–9) are great for training the cardiovascular system and you can also work on quick changes of direction.

Moderate leg strength will help speed and endurance as toned leg muscles can cope with higher demands of endurance. The Lunge, Knee Lift and Cross Chop (pp.50–51) takes the hip

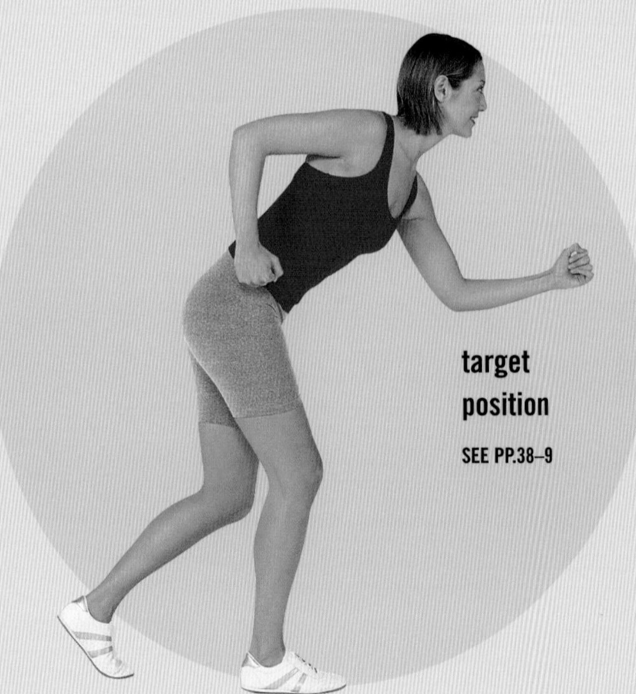

target position

SEE PP.38–9

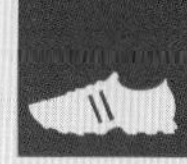

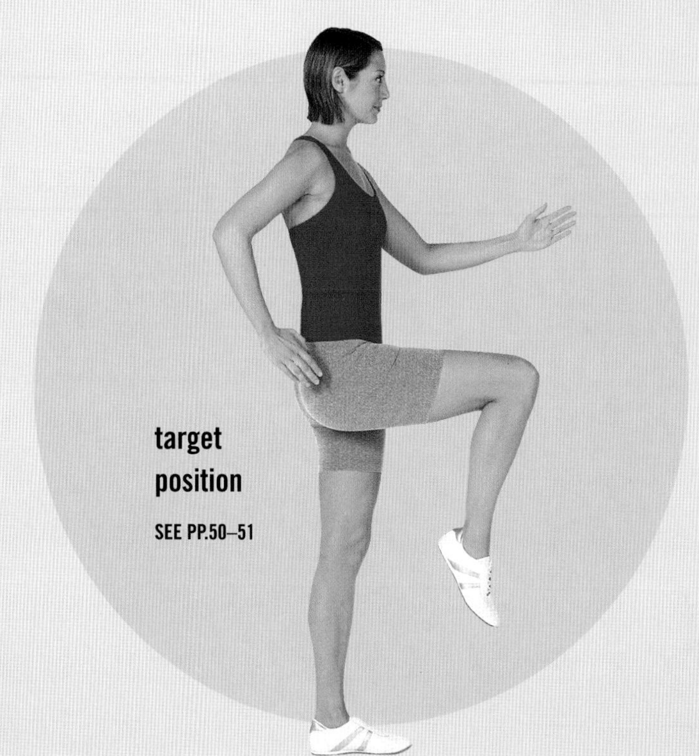

joint through a full range of movement, strengthens the legs and improves standing balance as well as synergy between the muscles around the hip, spine and pelvis.

Runners often develop short and tight hamstrings and hip flexor muscles, which can affect posture and body alignment. These muscles need to be stretched on a regular basis and after every session involving running (pp.66–7). The Gluts and Chest Stretch (pp.68–9) is another great stretch for runners. When you stretch you should not only work to maintain muscle length, you should also try to do developmental stretches. Hold the stretch until the muscle relaxes (30 to 60 seconds or longer), and then ease further into the stretch.

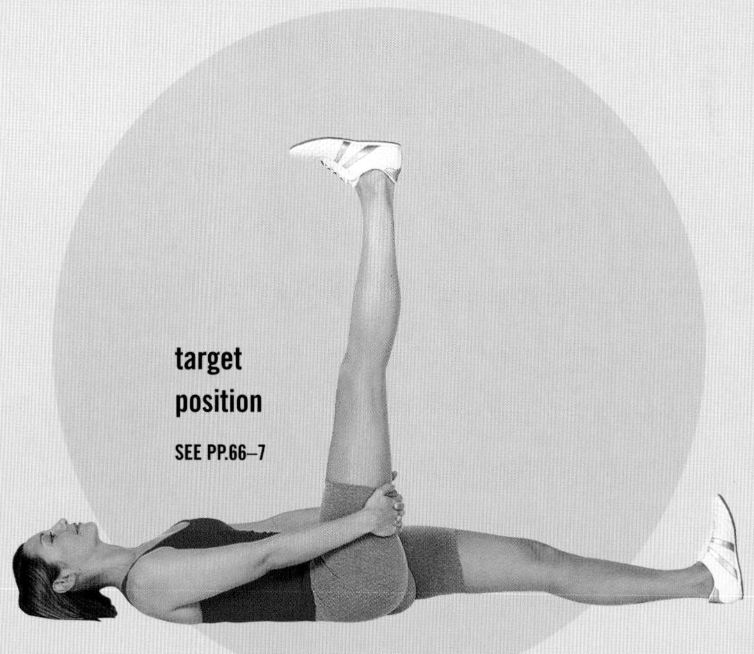

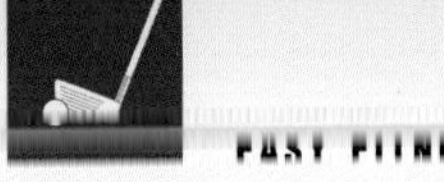

Easy fitness for golf

Golf is a game that relies on our rotational plane of movement. The golfer's body twists one way as he/she raises the golf club ready to take the shot, and twists the other way as the arms lower the club to hit the ball and follow through the shot. This is a dynamic movement involving speed, strength, flexibility and power through more than 180 degrees of rotation.

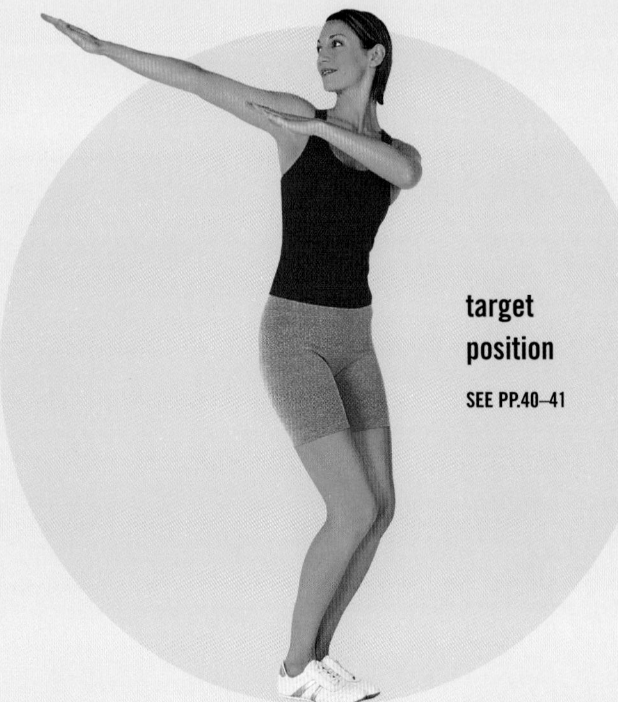

target position

SEE PP.40–41

The body is structured so that rotation can happen around the spine. We use rotational movements in daily life, for example, we might twist around to locate our seat belt in the car or to look through the rear windscreen as we park. In order to safely twist and avoid pulling a muscle, the body should be trained to switch on internal muscles to stabilize the core before the rotational movement occurs.

The Jumping Twists (pp.40–41) are ideal cardiovascular exercises that mimic the twisting movement at speed, and so dynamically train the oblique muscles that cause the twisting action. The Cross Chop arms

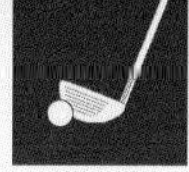

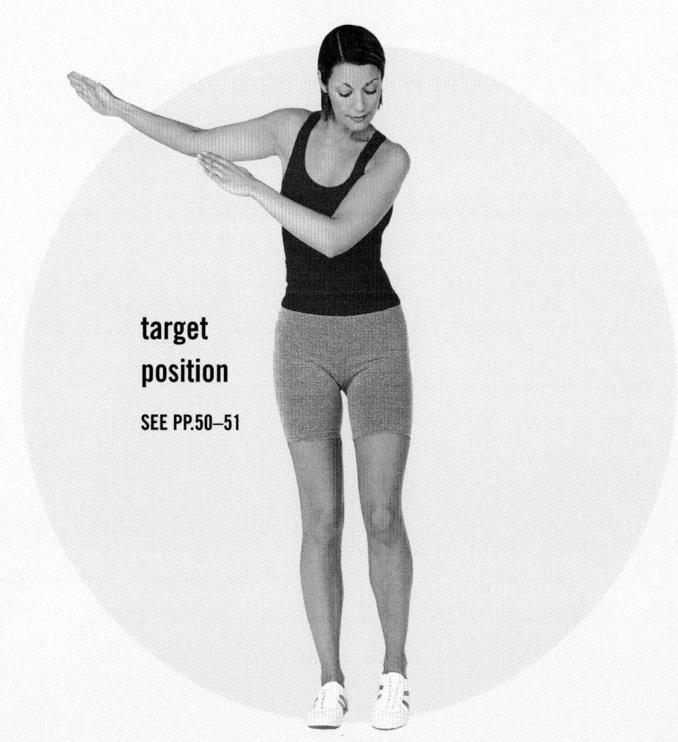

that accompany the Lunge (pp.50–51) are a good way of adding rotational movement to an exercise. The focus should be on slow, controlled movement to complement the faster pace of the Jumping Twists.

Combine these exercises with Back Extensions (pp.58–9), Prone Leg Lifts (pp.54–5), the Modified "T" Stand (pp.62–3), Press-ups (pp.56–7) and Tricep Dips (pp.52–3) to strengthen the back, chest and shoulders.

As the arms move together in a golf swing, you can modify the Lateral Stretch (pp.72–3) so that the arms reach away from each other to open and stretch through the chest. The Gluts and Chest Stretch (pp.68–9) is a good additional stretch.

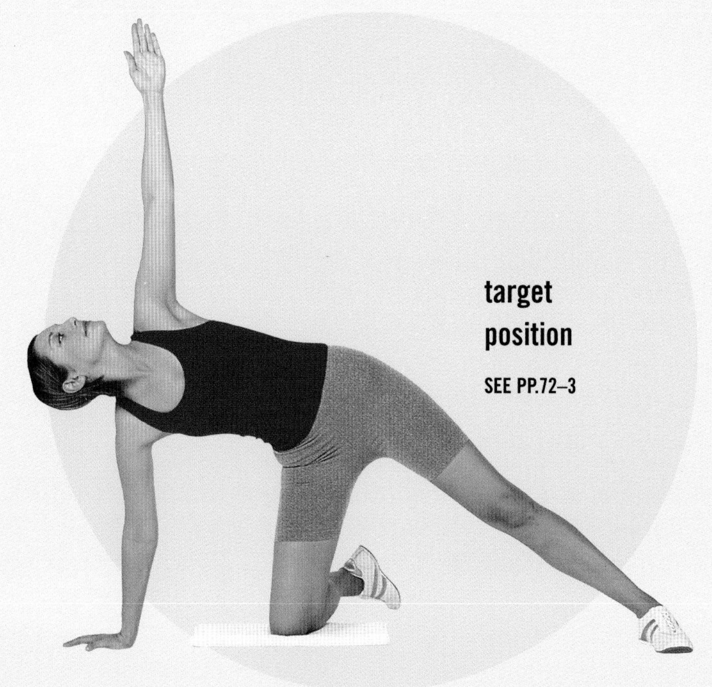

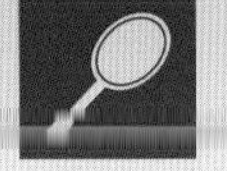

Easy fitness for racquet sports

We think of racquet sports, such as tennis and badminton, as demanding on the cardiovascular system, but they can also be quite intense on the hip, knee and ankle joints as most racquet sports involve a running and lunging action and require the ability to change direction quickly.

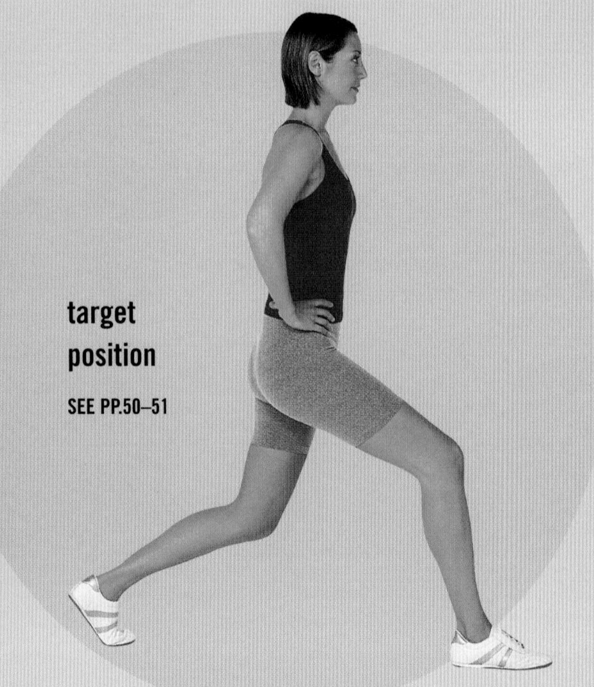

target position

SEE PP.50–51

The Sprint-runs (pp. 38–9) are excellent in terms of cardiovascular training. The exercise will help you improve speed and enable you to practise smooth changes of direction.

The Wall Jumps (pp.44–5) will help develop the player's ability to lift their body into the air to reach those high returns as well as improve joint stabilization on landing and moving. If you have problems with your hip, knee or ankle joints, try the heel raise solution (p.84).

The Lunges (pp.50–51) help prepare you to step into a space to take a shot, as well as lunging low to reach a low shot or one close to the net. You should do forward lunges, too.

Most racquet sports involve a forward leaning posture, but they also demand a lot of back strength as you move your shoulder back to take a regular shot or reach for a high shot. The back has to be strong yet mobile to avoid injuries. The Back Extension (pp.58–9) will help strengthen the back, the Bridge position (pp.64–5) will assist with mobilization and stabilization of the spine and the Cat Stretch (pp.74–5) will stretch out the back.

The running and lunging involved in racquet sports will especially work the gluteals. The chest muscles will also be constantly contracting as the racquet arm comes across the body. The combination Gluts and Chest Stretch (pp.68–9) is therefore an excellent stretch, but the racquet sport player will also benefit from all of the stretches in this book.

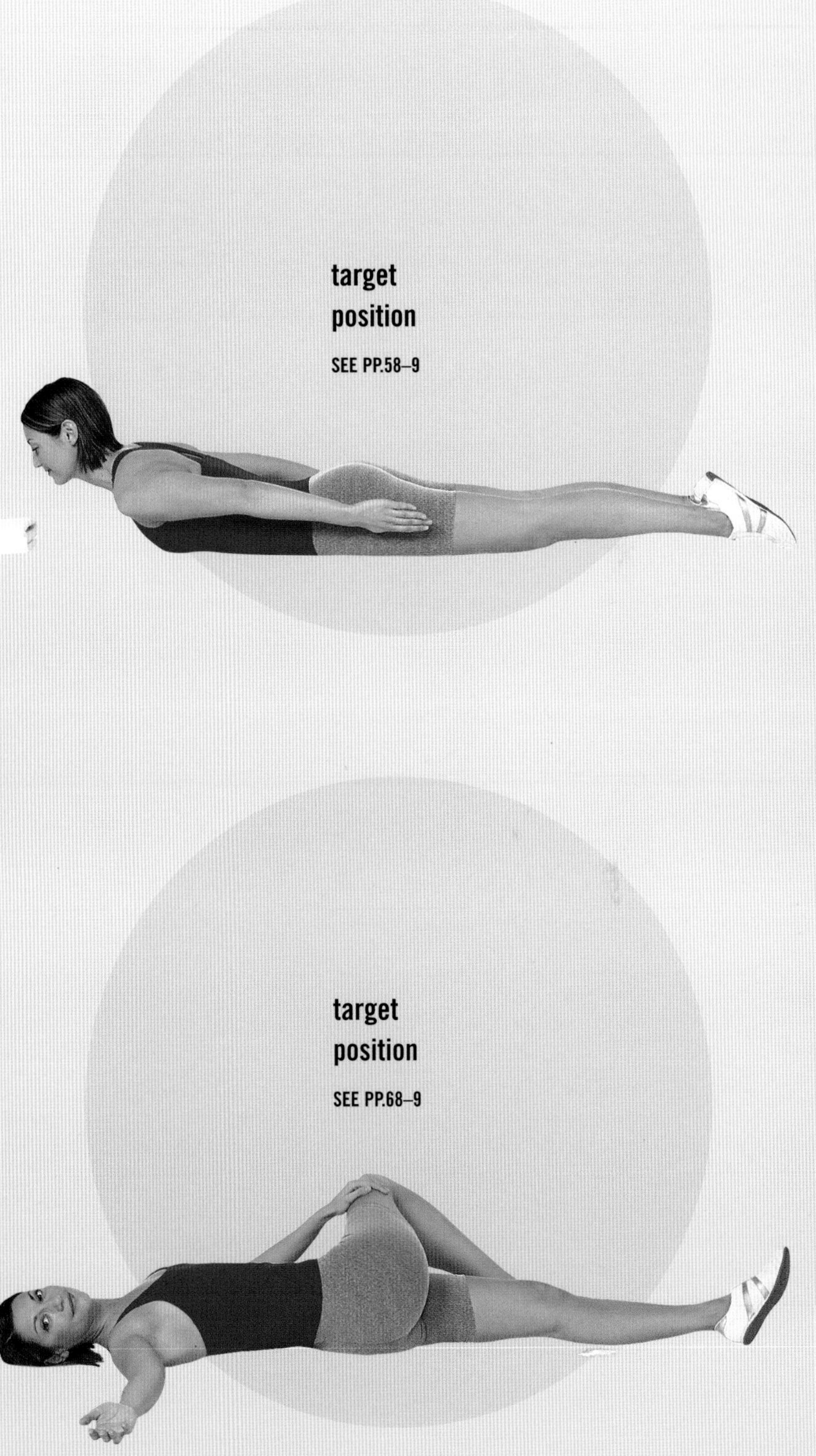

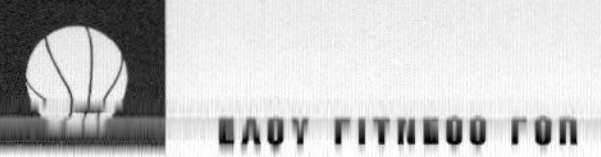

Easy fitness for ball sports

Ball sports, such as netball and basketball, demand speed and agility in addition to good levels of cardiovascular endurance. Players need to develop propulsion skills so that they can jump to shoot, catch and mark the ball.

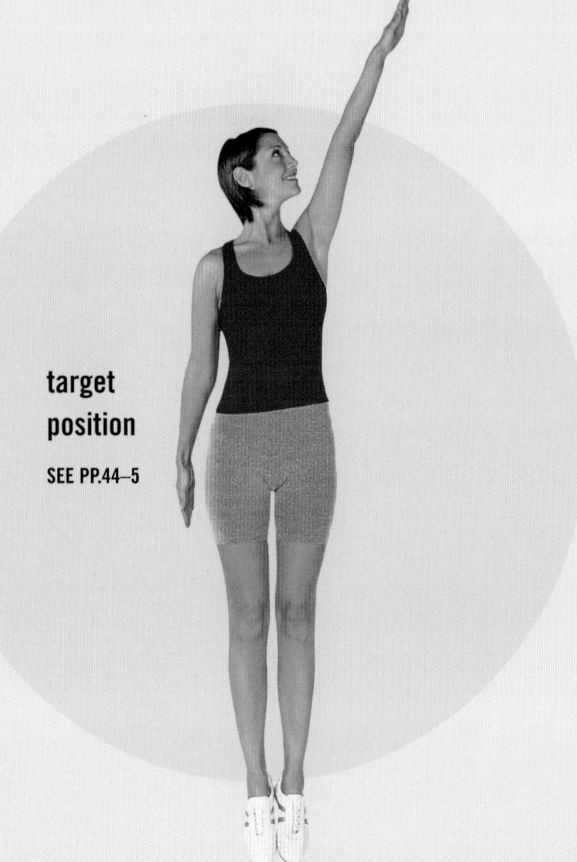

target position

SEE PP.44–5

The Wall Jumps (pp.44–5) work on jumping while moving and are great for preparing the ankle, knee and hip joints to execute a jump. Line Skiing (pp.46–7) and the Jumping Twists (pp.40–41) are also excellent exercises for ball sports. The combination of these three exercises will train all three planes of movement: sagittal (forward and backward); frontal (side to side); and transverse (twisting or rotating).

Strong, toned legs are required, not only to execute jumps but also for endurance, noting the length of a netball or basketball game. The Single Leg Squat (pp.48–9) strengthens the legs individually. This means that if one leg is weaker than the other, you can tailor your

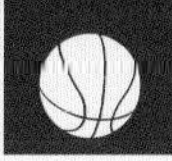

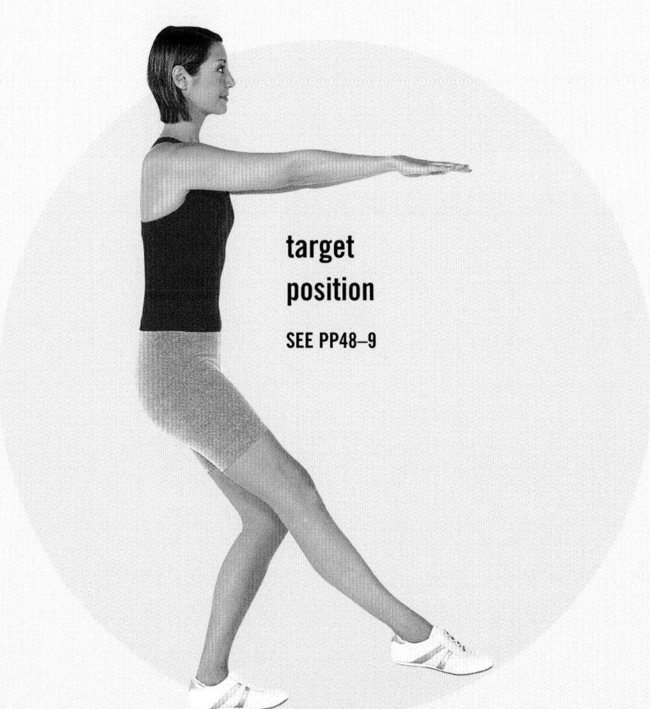

training to the strength of the weaker leg rather than always working to the strength of the stronger leg, and the imbalance between the right leg and left leg can be addressed. The exercise also improves balance, which is needed to enable the player to take off or land on one leg and still be balanced enough to make a good catch or throw.

The Lunge combination (pp.50–51) and Prone Leg Lift (pp.54–5) will strengthen the gluteals, quadriceps and hamstrings – the muscles involved in jumping.

Your after-session stretching should include a gluteal stretch such as the Gluts and Chest Stretch (pp.68–9) as well as stretches for the legs, chest, upper and lower back.

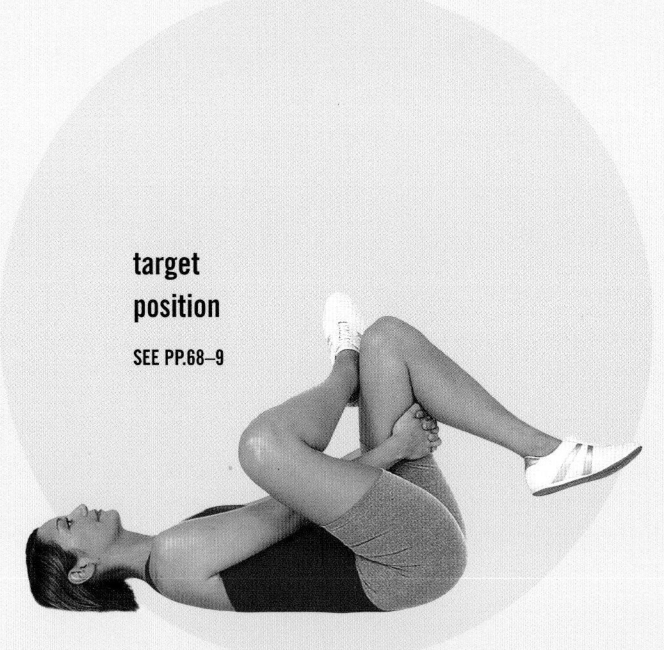

Easy fitness for combat sports

Both martial arts and boxing require upper body mobility and strength to punch, block and strike. Muscular endurance and agility of the legs and feet is needed for you to "go the distance", be light on your feet and dodge your opponent. Core strength is vital as the power behind any punch or kick comes from the centre of the body and travels out to the limbs.

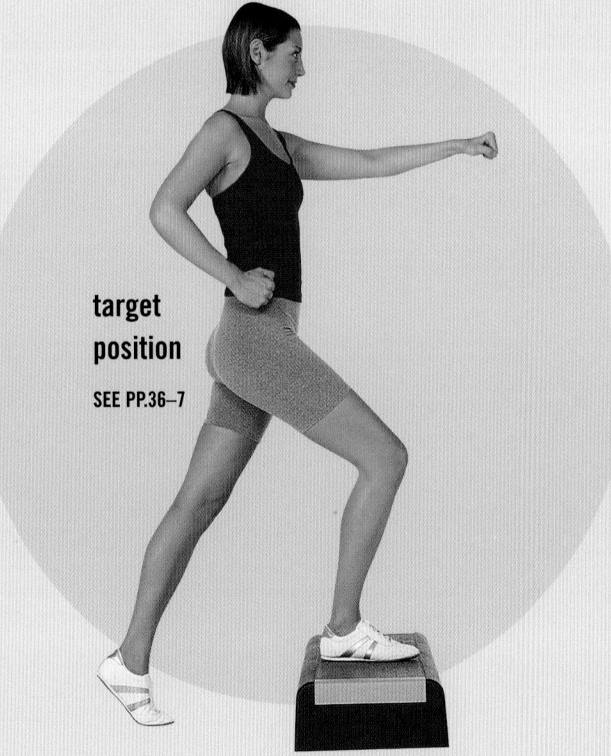

target position

SEE PP.36–7

Step-ups (pp.36–7) can be done to target cardiovascular training. You can heighten the intensity by increasing the speed at which you step. The exercise can even be done at more of a running pace as long as you can do this safely. When stepping at a slower pace, you can practise punches with your arms instead of doing the Chest Press. The Line Skiing (pp.46–7), Sprint-runs (pp.38–9) and Knee Lifts (pp.42–3) will also be of particular benefit.

The Press-ups (pp.56–7) will address upper body strength. A Press-up simultaneously stresses the wrist, elbow and shoulder joints, which can improve joint integrity and the way muscles around the joints work together. Closed chain movements (where the hands are connected to an immovable surface, such as the floor) load the joints in a way that an open chain movement (such as a bicep curl) cannot. A mixture of open chain and closed chain movements should be done in any training situation for optimal results. Single Leg Squats (pp.48–9), Lunges (pp.50–51), Modified “T” Stand (pp.62–3) and Back Extension (pp.58–9) should strengthen the legs and torso.

The Side-Lying Quad Stretch (pp.70–71) will stretch out the quadriceps after doing combat sports. The chest, hamstrings and hip flexors also need stretching, especially if you have done a lot of kicking in a martial arts session.

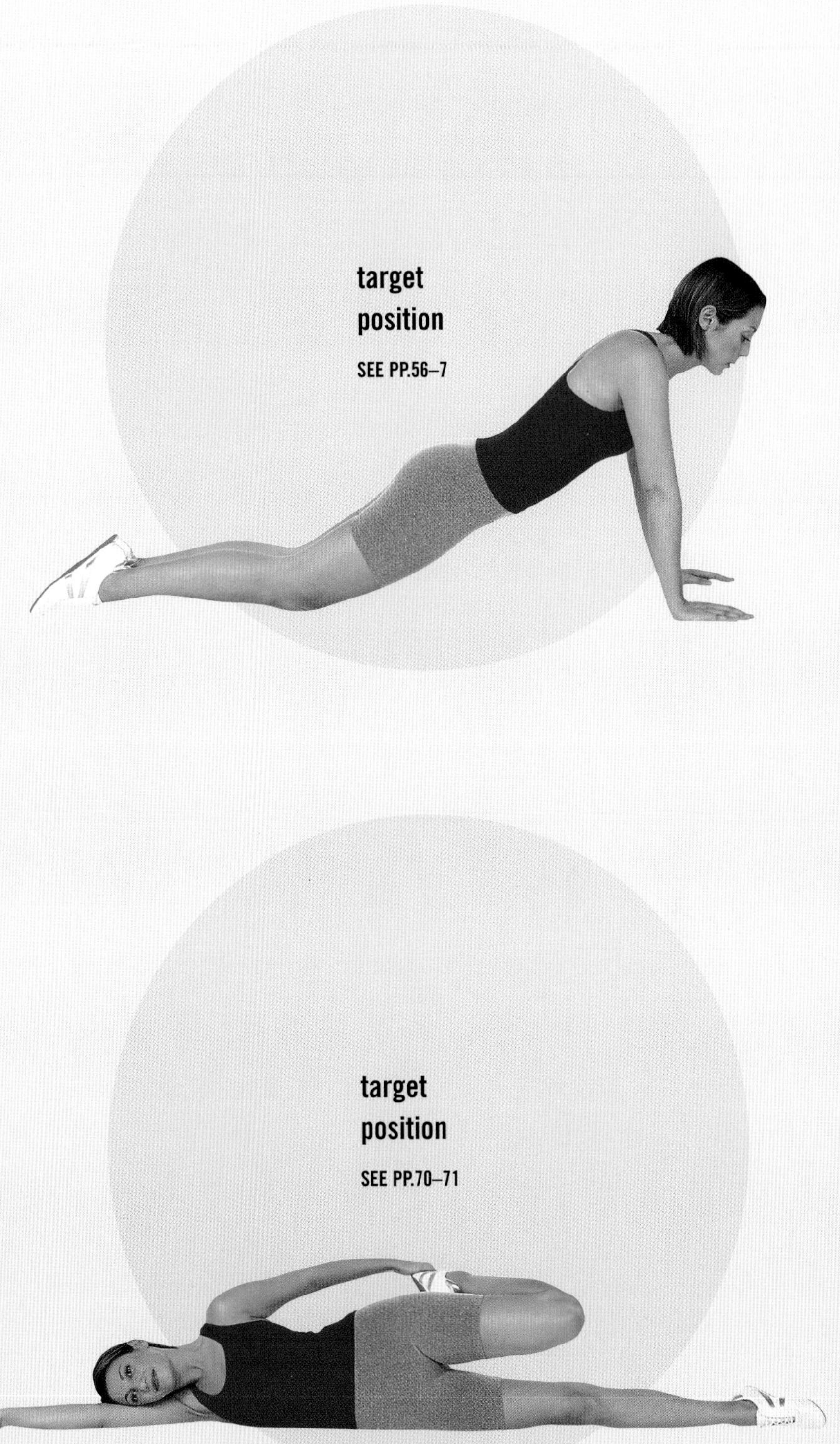

target position

SEE PP.56–7

target position

SEE PP.70–71

Bibliography

Blahnik, Jay *Full-body Flexibility*, Human Kinetics (Leeds, UK), 2004

Brittenham, Dean and Greg *Stronger Abs and Back*, Human Kinetics (Leeds, UK), 1997

Brooks, Douglas S. *Program Design for Personal Trainers*, Human Kinetics (Mammoth Lakes, CA), 1991

Fraser, Tara *The Easy Yoga Workbook*, Duncan Baird Publishers (London) and Thorsons (New York), 2003

Malcolm, Lorna Lee and Bender, Mark *Tone Yourself: Stretching for Health and Flexibility*, Duncan Baird Publishers (London), 1996 and Barnes & Noble (New York) 2000

McArdle, William D., Katch, Frank I. and Victor L. *Exercise Physiology: Energy, Nutrition and Human Performance* (third edition), Lea & Febiger (Philadelphia, US), 1998

Nash, Roscoe *Total Stretch*, MQ Publications (London), 2003

Norris, Christopher M. *Abdominal Training: Enhancing Core Stability* (second edition), A & C Black (London), 2001

Reebok University Programming Manuals, Reebok University Press (Toronto), (various dates)

Smith, Karen *The Easy Stretching Workbook*, Duncan Baird Publishers (London) and Thorsons (New York), 2004

Trew, Marion and Everett, Tony (Editors) *Human Movement: An Introductory Text* (fourth edition), Churchill Livingstone (Edinburgh, UK), 2001

Index

Page numbers in **bold** type refer to the main exercises.

Acknowledgments

I would like to thank Julia Charles at Duncan Baird Publishers (who first approached me with the idea) and Justin Ford, Zoë Stone and the rest of the creative team at DBP. Matthew Ward (photographer) was ever the professional and so easy to work with. I need to thank Hanna Curtis who modelled for this book and was always cheerful and willing to repeat a move, even the jumps, as many times as it took with no complaints! I would also like to thank hair and make-up artist Tinks Reding. Lastly, I would like to acknowledge Reebok and Pure Energy for sponsoring and supporting me within the fitness industry for so many years and my family who are always there to support and never cease to show me their love. Thank you.